# The Encyclopedia of Herbal Medicine for Pets: 300+ Natural Remedies to Promote Wellness in Dogs, Cats, Horses & Exotic Animals.

Subtitle: Harnessing Nature's Healing Power for Your Beloved Pets

By

**Lily Green**

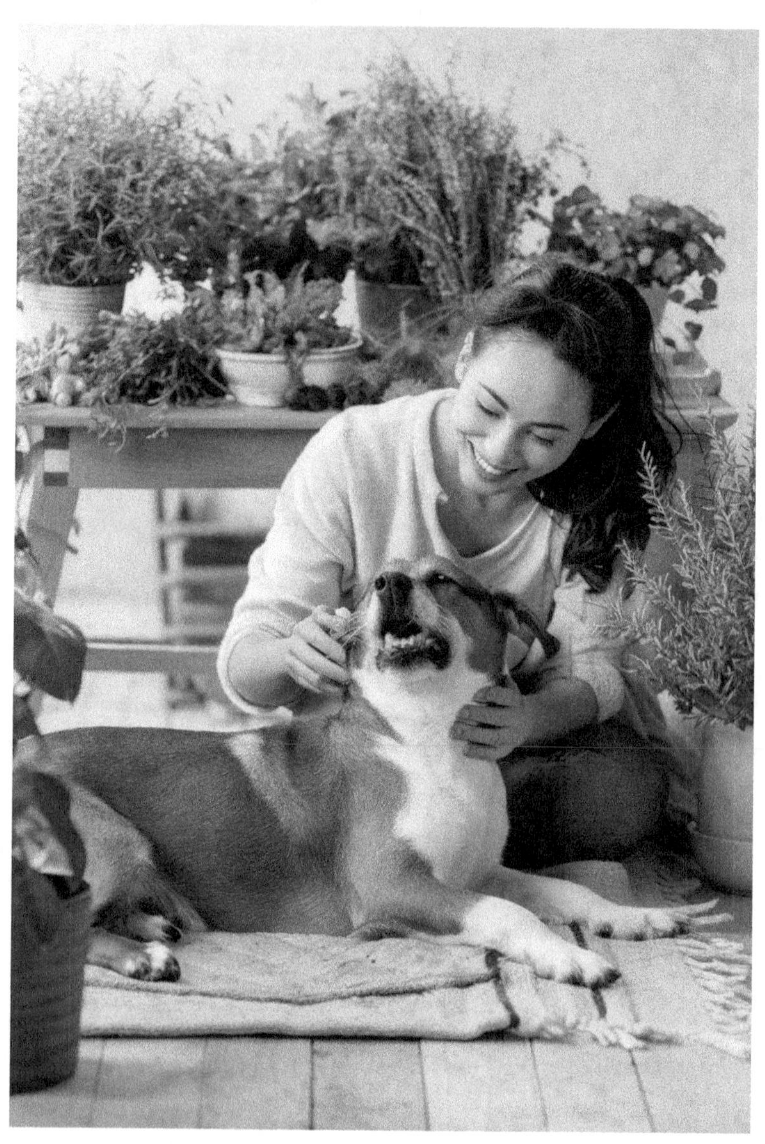

# Chapter Outlines:

## Preface

The human-animal bond is a powerful and enduring force. Our pets offer us unconditional love, companionship, and a unique form of emotional support. In return, we strive to provide them with a life filled with love, happiness, and optimal health.

For centuries, various cultures around the world have harnessed the power of plants to promote human well-being. This very same wisdom holds immense potential for our animal companions. **The Encyclopedia of Herbal Medicine for Pets** delves into this fascinating realm, offering a comprehensive exploration of natural remedies for dogs, cats, horses, and even exotic animals.

This book is not intended as a substitute for professional veterinary advice. Always consult with your veterinarian before introducing any new remedies into your pet's routine. However, it aspires to empower you with knowledge and equip you to explore the potential benefits of herbal medicine in collaboration with your veterinarian.

As you embark on this journey, remember that the most crucial ingredient in your pet's healthcare journey is love. This book serves as a guide, but your unwavering love and devotion are the foundation of your pet's well-being.

**Forward**

Imagine a world where nature's bounty becomes a valuable tool in nurturing the health of your beloved pet. A world where ancient wisdom merges with modern veterinary knowledge to create a holistic approach to animal wellness. **The Encyclopedia of Herbal Medicine for Pets** brings this vision to life.

Within these pages, you'll discover a treasure trove of information on herbal remedies specifically tailored to various animal companions. From the playful antics of a canine friend to the majestic grace of a horse, this book caters to the unique needs of each species.

Whether you're a seasoned pet owner or just beginning your journey, this encyclopedia offers valuable insights and practical guidance. It empowers you to ask informed questions, explore natural solutions with your veterinarian, and become a proactive advocate for your pet's health.

As a veterinarian with a deep passion for both traditional and complementary approaches to animal care, I'm thrilled to introduce you to this resource. **The Encyclopedia of Herbal Medicine for Pets** is not a magic bullet, but it's a valuable addition to your pet's healthcare library. Let it guide you on a path of discovery, fostering a deeper connection with your pet and nurturing their well-being with the wisdom of nature.

# Dr.Lily Green.

## Dedication

*To all the devoted pet owners who cherish the bond they share with their furry (or feathered) companions. May this book empower you to become a champion for their health and well-being, nurturing their vitality with the gentle touch of nature?*

# Chapter 1

# Introduction to Herbal Medicine for Pets

Does your furry (or feathered) companion deserve a life filled with vibrant health and happiness? Do you yearn to explore natural approaches to complement your pet's well-being? Look no further than **The Encyclopedia of Herbal Medicine for Pets**! This comprehensive guide unlocks the secrets of the plant world, empowering you to become a proactive advocate for your pet's health.

Within these pages, you'll embark on a transformative journey, discovering over

300 natural remedies tailored to a variety of animal companions. Whether you share your life with a loyal dog, a mischievous cat, a majestic horse, or an exotic friend, this encyclopedia offers a wealth of knowledge specifically designed for their unique needs.

Forget about generic information – delve into targeted herbal solutions for dogs, cats, horses, and even exotic animals! This isn't just a collection of remedies; it's a treasure trove of insights into using nature's pharmacy to nurture your pet's vitality.

**Here's a glimpse of the enriching exploration that awaits you:**

- **Understanding the Power of Plants:** Gain a foundational understanding of herbal medicine and its potential benefits for promoting pet wellness.

- **A Species-Specific Approach:** Uncover targeted herbal remedies tailored to the unique physiological needs of dogs, cats, horses, and exotic animals.

- **300+ Natural Solutions:** Explore a comprehensive library of herbal remedies for a wide range of health concerns, from digestive issues to anxiety and beyond.

- **Safety First:** Learn crucial safety guidelines for administering herbal remedies and potential herb-drug interactions to ensure your pet's well-being.

- **Holistic Harmony:** Discover how to integrate herbal medicine with conventional veterinary care to create a well-rounded approach to your pet's health.

**The Encyclopedia of Herbal Medicine for Pets** is more than just a book; it's a testament to the deep connection we share with our animal companions. It's a bridge between ancient wisdom and modern veterinary knowledge, empowering you to nurture your pet's health naturally. Are you ready to unlock the secrets of nature's healing power for your beloved pet? Let's begin!

# Chapter 2 - Herbs for Skin and Coat Health

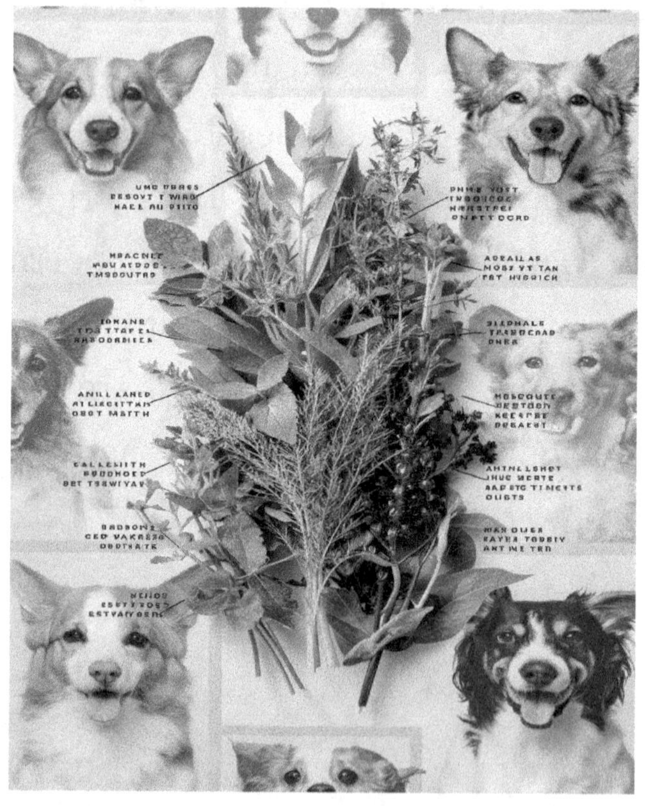

As an attentive pet parent, you've probably noticed how intricately connected your furry friend's skin and coat condition are to their overall wellness. After all, the skin is the body's largest organ, acting as a protective barrier while also allowing vital processes like temperature regulation and toxin removal. When skin health is compromised, it can manifest in irritating, unsightly, and sometimes painful ways - from dry, flaky dandruff to hot spots and dermatitis.

Luckily, Mother Nature has gifted us with an array of botanicals that can help soothe, protect, and optimize your pet's skin and coat from the inside out. In this chapter, we'll explore some of the top herbal remedies and preparations for nurturing healthy skin and fur. Get ready to harness the power of nature's healing herbs for your pet's utmost comfort and radiance!

## The Skin and Coat's Important Functions

Before we dive into herbal solutions, let's first appreciate why maintaining healthy skin is so vital for your animal companion's wellbeing:

- **Barrier Protection:** The outer skin layers create a physical barrier that shields the body from environmental threats like chemicals, microbes, injuries, and UV radiation.

- **Temperature Regulation:** Hair follicles play a key role in insulation and heat regulation through panting, sweating, and piloerection (fur sticking up).

- **Immune Function:** The skin contains immune cells that help recognize and fight off pathogens and irritants.

- **Sensation:** Numerous nerve endings allow the skin to transmit sensations like touch, pain, pressure, and temperature across the body.

- **Excretion:** Sweat glands and sebaceous glands remove waste products and excessive hormones from the body through the skin.

- **Appearance:** For many pets, healthy skin, and a lustrous coat boosts confidence and physical appeal.

When skin health suffers due to allergies, infections, hormonal changes, or nutritional deficiencies, it impacts the entire body's equilibrium. Using gentle herbs that respect the skin's integral roles can restore balance.

## The Power of Botanical Skin Soothers

Nature offers an array of botanicals that provide targeted herbal support for various skin and coat concerns. Let's take a look at some top plant allies for common dermatological issues:

### Calendula

Among herbalists, this sunny orange flower is considered the preeminent skin herb.

Calendula's Anti-inflammatory, antimicrobial, and antioxidant properties make it a multipurpose healer for all kinds of dermatological woes:

- **Skin Irritations** - The flavonoids in calendula help reduce inflammation, swelling, and itchiness from rashes, dermatitis, and allergies. Its wound-healing abilities help skin recover quickly.

- **Hot Spots** - Calendula soothes those angry, red, moist skin lesions that pets incessantly lick and chew by fighting infection and promoting fast tissue repair.

- **Wounds/Ulcers** - This herb helps disinfect cuts, abrasions,s and pressure sores while stimulating new tissue growth for faster recovery.

**- Colitis/Anal Gland Issues -** Calendula can be used in sitz baths or compresses to bring relief for inflamed anal glands and rectal irritations.

The vibrant orange hue comes from carotenoid antioxidants, which help strengthen skin against environmental stressors like UV damage. Calendula is gentle enough for regular use on sensitive areas.

## Chamomile

This daisy-like flower herb has rightfully earned a reputation as one of the most versatile herbs in skin care. With anti-inflammatory, anti-allergenic, antiseptic, and antioxidant properties, chamomile proves invaluable:

- **Dermatitis** - Chamomile helps reduce redness, irritation, and itchiness associated with allergic dermatitis and eczema flare-ups.

- **Hot Spots** - Applying a chamomile compress can quickly calm inflamed "hot spots" and fight off secondary bacterial or yeast infections.

- **Wounds/Burns** - Used topically, chamomile's antimicrobial azulene compounds help disinfect and regenerate damaged skin tissues.

**- Irritated Eyes -** Chamomile eye washes alleviate redness, styes, weepy eyes, and conjunctivitis thanks to its anti-inflammatory effects.

**- Ear Conditions -** It helps soothe outer ear inflammation and infections when used as a rinse.

**- Anxiety-Related Skin Issues -** The light sedative properties in chamomile can help pets who compulsively lick, chew, or over groom due to stress/anxiety.

Both German (***Matricaria recutita***) and Roman (***Chamaemelum nobile***) chamomile offer skin-friendly benefits. The dried flowers make a wonderful base for healing herbal salves and skin rinses.

## Aloe Vera

You may already have this succulent "burn plant" in your home! Aloe's cooling gel provides near-instant topical relief backed by anti-inflammatory compounds:

- **Dermal Burns** - Whether from fire, chemicals, or extreme sun exposure, aloe helps improve healing time while reducing pain and the probability of scarring.

- **Wounds/Abrasions** - Rich in glycoproteins and polysaccharides, the gel encourages faster skin regeneration on cuts, scrapes, bites, and hot spots.

- **Boo-Boo Remedy** - For stings, minor burns, scratches, or localized inflammations, just snip an aloe leaf and apply the fresh gel directly.

## - Coat Conditioner -

Aloe is an amazing ingredient for hydrating and soothing inflamed, sunburned, or irritated skin. The rich nutrient profile promotes faster tissue repair. When used liberally, it creates a protective barrier against environmental stressors.

## Oatmeal

Humble oats pack a surprising punch when it comes to calming enraged skin. From topical baths and rinses to oral supplements, oatmeal delivers:

- **Anti-Irritant Properties** - Compounds called avenanthramides reduce redness, itchiness, and inflammation associated with dermatitis flare-ups.

- **Gentle Cleansing** - Saponins give oats a natural soap-like lather for cleansing without stripping natural skin oils.

- **Moisturizing Effects** - Proteins and lipids present in oats create a conditioning barrier to seal in hydration.

- **Nutrients** - Oats supply skin-nourishing vitamins (B, E), antioxidants (ferulic acid), and vital fatty acids for healthy tissues.

Ground into a fine powder, oatmeal can be stirred into bath water for full-body soaks, dusted on as a dry shampoo, or applied as a soothing paste for irritated spots. The gentle action makes it safe for puppies and kittens.

**Neem**

This little evergreen tree holds a big skin-saving power! Found frequently in Ayurvedic medicine, neem treats various dermatological issues:

- **Anti-Parasitic** - Neem seed oil contains over 60 antiparasitic compounds effective against fleas, mites, ticks, ringworm, and other topical pests.

- **Antibacterial/Antifungal** - Rich in flavonoids and antimicrobials that fight skin infections like hot spots, bacterial pyoderma, and candidiasis.

- **Anti-Inflammatory** - Helps ease itchiness, pain and inflammation involved in allergic dermatitis and other skin irritations.

- **Purifying** - Astringent properties allow neem to dry up oozing sores and blemishes while promoting faster healing.

Neem oil smells a bit nutty and bitter, but only temporarily when applied to skin or coats. Use it as an insect repellent spray, shampoo additive, or spot treatment. Just avoid getting it near eyes, noses, or open wounds.

## Tea Tree Oil

Don't let the "tree" part fool you - this powerful extract comes from an Australian shrub and makes a superb antifungal/antibacterial treatment:

**- Yeast/Fungal Issues** - Tea tree oil takes the cake when fighting stubborn yeast infections, ringworm, and other fungal conditions on skin and nails.

**- Ear Infections** - Diluted tea tree oil helps fight fungal and bacterial ear infections in the outer ear canal when used properly.

**- Hot Spots:** - Thanks to its antiseptic action, tea trees help halt the spread of infection in hot spots and abrasions.

**- Dandruff/Seborrhea** - This oil helps normalize excessive sebum production and clear up scaly, flaky skin.

A little goes a long way with potent tea tree oil, making proper dilution critical to avoid irritation. Use as a spot treatment, mix into shampoo, or combine with a carrier oil for massage or dips.

**Herbal Shampoos and Rinses**

While a high-quality pet shampoo certainly has merits, many contain harsh surfactants that strip away precious skin oils. Herbal shampoos and rinses offer a gentler, moisturizing alternative for grooming your pet while imparting vital skin-nourishing benefits.

We'll start with a basic gentle recipe suitable for weekly bathing or as an in-between rinse for dogs, cats, and other furry companions.

This blend incorporates some of the soothing herbs we just covered:

**Colloidal Oatmeal & Chamomile Bath Supplies:**

- 1 cup colloidal oatmeal (finely ground whole oats)
- 1/4 cup dried chamomile flowers
- Muslin herb bag or tied cheesecloth
- 1 gallon hot water

**Instructions:**

1. Place oats and chamomile into the muslin bag/tied cheesecloth bundle and secure.
2. In a clean bucket or sink, pour the hot water over the herb bundle and allow it to steep for 20-30 minutes to extract botanical properties.

3. Prepare your pet's bath using warm water as normal. Submerse and swish the herb bundle thoroughly to release the oils and nutrients into the bath.

4. Bathe your pet with the herbal-infused water, allowing them to soak for 5-10 minutes before rinsing. Gently squeeze more liquid from the herb bundle as needed.

5. Follow with a light coating of aloe vera gel as a leave-in conditioner before drying.

This gentle blend helps cleanse while moisturizing and imparting chamomile's anti-inflammatory and antimicrobial effects to soothe irritation. The oatmeal creates a milky, colloidal suspension that helps seal in hydration. Perfect for sensitive skin! Let's explore a few more targeted herbal shampoo recipes:

**Neem Oil Anti-Pest Shampoo:**

¼ cup neem seed oil

¼ cup colloidal oatmeal

1 tbsp aloe vera gel

8 oz unscented mild shampoo

Combine all ingredients thoroughly. Work deeply into the coat, let sit for 5-10 mins, then rinse. Offers long-lasting insect repellent protection.

**Baking Soda and Herbs Dry Shampoo:**
¼ cup baking soda

¼ cup dried rosemary

2 tbsp dried lavender flowers

Grind into a fine powder using a blender or coffee grinder. Rub directly into the dry coat, let sit for 10 mins, then brush out thoroughly. Great for deodorizing and freshening coats between baths.

## Herbal Salves and Spot Treatments

For localized areas of skin irritation, inflammation or infection, herbal salves make the perfect treatment to speed healing. When infused with skin-repairing botanicals, salves create an antimicrobial, hydrating barrier while providing pain relief.

The basic process involves combining dried herbs with a high-quality carrier oil like olive, sweet almond or jojoba. This allows the beneficial phytochemicals and nutrients to become dissolved and concentrated in the oil through heated infusion.

Once the herbs have released their properties into the infused oil, beeswax or plant-derived wax gets blended in to create the smooth, spreadable ointment consistency. Here's a multi-purpose herbal salve perfect for hot spots, cuts, rashes, dry skin and more:

**Botanical Skin Repair Salve**
**Supplies:**

- 1 cup calendula flowers, dried
- 1/4 cup plantain leaf, dried
- 1/4 cup comfrey leaf, dried
- 1 cup olive, almond or jojoba oil
- 1/2 oz beeswax pellets
- 10-15 drops lavender essential oil (optional)

**Instructions:**

1. In a double boiler or heat-proof glass bowl, combine the dried herbs and oil. Place this bowl into a pan filled with 1-2 inches of water.

2. Gently heat the oil/herb mixture for 30-60 minutes, keeping the temperature around 100F - never boiling. This allows the botanical properties to fully infuse into the oil.

3. Strain out the herbs from the infused oil using a mesh strainer or muslin bag. Squeeze well to extract all the liquid.

4. Return the infused oil to a double boiler and warm over low heat. Add in the beeswax pellets and allow to fully melt, stirring frequently.

5. Once uniform and liquefied, remove from heat and stir in lavender oil if using.

6. Carefully pour the herbal salve into sterilized tins or jars and allow to fully cool before applying lids.

To use: Gently massage the salve into affected skin areas 1-3 times daily after cleansing. Reapply as needed until condition resolves. The antibacterial, anti-inflammatory, and soothing effects will get to work!

For stubborn conditions like ringworm or yeast infections, feel free to bolster your salve with antifungal powerhouses like tea tree, oregano, and neem:

**Anti-Fungal Herbal Salve**

Follow the basic salve instructions above, but add these ingredients:
- ½ cup tea tree essential oil
- ¼ cup oregano leaf
- ¼ cup neem leaf

Of course, there are countless botanical combinations to experiment with based on your pet's particular coat and skin conditions. Let your intuition guide you, and have fun creating customized herbal salves!

## Hydrosols and Sprays

For an easy, mess-free solution to itchy skin and pest prevention, whipping up a hydrosol spray makes life simpler. You'll just need to collect the fragrant-waters created during the steam distillation of botanicals.

This process concentrates the gentle, water-soluble portions of an herb or floral essence into an aromatic liquid filled with trace nutrients, enzymes, and active compounds. So while not as potent as essential oils, hydrosols offer subtler benefits:

- Calming mild skin irritations, rashes, hot spots
- Relieving itchiness and inflammation
- Deterring pests like fleas and ticks
- Conditioning and deodorizing coats
- Perfect for frequent, mess-free application

One of the most multifaceted hydrosols is derived from the roses:

**Rose Hydrosol Skin Spray**

Ingredients:

- 8 oz rose hydrosol (or rose petal water)

- 2 oz witch hazel extract

- 5 drops vitamin E oil

- 10 drops rose geranium essential oil (optional)

## Directions:

1. In a spray bottle, combine all ingredients and swirl gently to integrate.

2. Mist directly onto irritated skin areas, hot spots, dry patches, or the full coat.

3. Allow to air dry. No rinsing required.

4. Reapply as needed throughout the day.

The naturally cooling and anti-inflammatory properties of rose hydrosol soothe itchy, inflamed skin. Witch hazel acts as an astringent to help dry up oozing areas. Rose geranium oil lends extra antibacterial effects.

Here's another simple spray that makes good use of that ultra-soothing herb, chamomile:

## Chamomile & Aloe Hydrating Spritz
**Ingredients:**
- 8 oz chamomile hydrosol
- 2 oz aloe vera juice
- 2 tsp vegetable glycerine

**Directions:**
1. Combine all ingredients in a spray bottle. No need for essential oils here.
2. Mist over dry, irritated skin and brushed-out fur as needed, concentrating on problem areas.

3. Towel-dry pet after application if desired, but no rinsing required.

4. Great for spritzing on hotspots, dry noses and paws to rehydrate and soothe.

The beauty of these sprays lies in their versatility. They hydrate and heal while imparting coat sheen and pleasant aromatics that lightly repel bugs. Mist your pet as often as needed - before walks, after baths, or anytime to reset their coat.

Absolutely, I'm happy to continue expanding on this chapter about using herbs for optimal skin and coat health in pets:

## Building Your Herbal First Aid Kit

Every pet owner should keep a few key herbal preparations on hand for those inevitable scratches, rashes, and skin irritations that crop up. Here are some must-have botanical allies to stock:

**Calendula Tincture**

Calendula's skin-healing, antimicrobial properties make this tincture a multi-purpose first aid hero. Use it to:
- Disinfect cuts, abrasions, and wounds by applying directly
- Soothe itchy rashes and dermatitis by adding to a spray bottle with water
- Ease angry hot spots by spritzing on the irritated area several times daily
- Support healing after surgery by applying along incision sites

## Activated Charcoal

This black powder may look unremarkable, but it's a powerful absorptive agent. Mix with a bit of water or aloe gel to create a paste for:

- Drawing out insect stings, splinters, and snake bites
- Absorbing bacterial toxins from wounds and infections
- Relieving gas/bloating when administered orally in small amounts

## Green Clay

Rich in minerals, this cosmetic clay becomes a versatile base for soothing poultices:

- Mix with calendula tincture or hydrosol into a spreadable paste

- Apply directly to hot spots, abscesses, and insect bites to draw out toxins
- Let dry fully before rinsing - the clay will harden as it pulls out impurities

**Herbal Salve**

An herbal salve like the recipes provided earlier offers deep, penetrating healing for:
- Cuts, abrasions, and surgical wound sites
- Cracked paw pads, dry noses and elbows
- Dandruff, dermatitis, and other inflammatory skin conditions

**Essential Oil Blends**

Properly diluted essential oil blends serve many skin and coat care purposes, including:
- Anti-itch relief for allergic dermatitis, flea bites

- Antimicrobial barriers against bacterial/fungal infections
- Insect repellent sprays when misted over coat before going outdoors
- Aromatherapy calming effects to curb licking/chewing behaviors

Be sure to only purchase quality oils from reputable suppliers and use extreme caution with proper dilution rates for each oil.

Keeping an assortment of these herbal skin care basics in your pet's medical kit ensures you'll be prepared to offer immediate, natural relief and accelerated healing.

## Nutrition's Role in Skin Health

You may have noticed that many skin issues first arise due to an underlying dietary deficiency or imbalance. An inappropriate diet lacking quality proteins, vitamins, minerals, and essential fatty acids can manifest as dull coats, dry skin, hot spots, and a host of dermatological problems.

Luckily, there are some fantastic skin/coat-boosting herbs you can incorporate into your pet's daily meals:

- **Nettles** - Rich in silica, nettles promote lustrous fur while reducing shedding. The anti-inflammatory nutrients also soothe allergic reactions.

- **Alfalfa** - A powerhouse of vitamins A, D, E, K plus trace minerals that nourish and regenerate skin from within.

- **Spirulina** - Concentrated protein and omega-3s help repair tissues and ease inflammation. The high antioxidant levels protect against environmental stressors.

- **Burdock Root** - Detoxifying compounds flush accumulated impurities from the bloodstream and tissues to clear skin irritations.

These herbs can be:
- Sprinkled in powder form over kibble or raw food

- Blended into homemade broths or dehydrated treat mixtures
- Given as concentrated herbal capsules or tinctures

My top tip? Brew an uber-nutritious herbal "tea" by steeping these dried herbs along with things like:

- Dandelion leaf and root
- Yellow dock root
- Milk thistle seed
- Turmeric root

Then use the strained liquid as a nutritive food topper or drinking water base. This infuses meals with skin/coat-enriching vitamins, minerals and antioxidants.

Making Herbal Medicine Grooming Fun

I'll let you in on a little secret... giving your dog or cat their "herbal remedies" doesn't have to feel like a chore! With a bit of creativity, you can turn skin/coat care into a bonding routine you both enjoy.

For instance, does your pup go wild for a doggy massage? Combine it with the benefits of essential oil therapy by diluting a few drops of skin-nourishing oils like:

- Lavender - For calming itchy, inflamed skin
- Geranium - Balances oil production for less dandruff
- Cedarwood - Promotes thick, shiny coats and repels pests

- Frankincense - Soothes skin allergies and irritation

Into a carrier oil like fractionated coconut, then gently massage over their body while brushing out the coat. Your dog will be in seventh heaven!

Or pamper your fastidious feline with a DIY clay mask using:

- Bentonite, rhassoul, or french green clay
- Hydrosols like rose, chamomile, or lavender water
- A dollop of aloe vera gel

Mix into a luxurious paste, then gently spread over your kitty's face and body while giving loving pets and scratches. Let the minerals and botanicals work magic, then rinse off the mask for silky fur.

See what I mean? Caring for your pet's skin and coat doesn't have to be all business. By combining therapeutic herbs and oils with the very things your animal adores - massage, grooming, play - you turn treatment into fun, bonding experiences.

Your pet will not only gain the benefits of beautiful skin, but their overall wellbeing will thrive as you strengthen that interspecies connection through affection and positive reinforcement. Baths, spot treatments, and medicines don't have to be a battle - they can actually become cherished rituals.

So get creative! Explore different herbal-infused grooming tools, spritzes, balms and playtime remedies. With a little herbal ingenuity, you and your pet will look forward to spa days in no time.

I hope this chapter has opened your eyes to the incredible botanical support system available for nurturing radiant skin and lustrous coats. Like any new therapy, start slowly while closely monitoring how your pet responds. With patience and your veterinarian's guidance, these time-honored herbal remedies can work gently yet powerfully to restore vibrance to your faithful companion.

Enjoy this blissful, earth-derived path to balanced dermatological health! Onward to the next chapter, where we explore how herbs can specifically benefit joints, mobility and age-related aches and pains. Your pet's overall wellness journey is just beginning.

# Chapter 3 - Joint and Mobility Support

Movement is life. Anyone who has witnessed a beautiful being confined to stillness due to joint issues understands just how crucial flexibility and ease of motion are to overall vitality and wellbeing. Our animal friends rely on their bodies' full range of motion not just for ambulation, but for core functions like grooming, playing, hunting, and even digesting food properly. Compromised joint health can severely diminish their quality of life.

Arthritis, hip and elbow dysplasia, intervertebral disk disease - these are just some of the common joint afflictions our beloved dogs, cats, rabbits, and other pets face, especially as they age. Repetitive injuries, conformational defects, excessive weight, and inflammation can all contribute to deteriorating joint structures over time. The resulting pain, loss of mobility, and muscle atrophy disrupt the very essence of what allows an animal to thrive.

The good news? A wide array of herbs offer natural support to preserve joint and musculoskeletal health in our animal companions. In this chapter, we'll explore key botanicals that reduce inflammation, lubricate joints, repair cartilage, and build strength and flexibility. You'll learn how to incorporate herbal supplements, topicals, and complementary therapies for a comprehensive joint care approach to keep your pet happy, pain-free and in motion.

## The Roles of Healthy Joints and Mobility

To better understand how herbs function in maintaining joint health, we first need to appreciate the brilliant design and mechanics that underlie our pets' ability to move and flex.

Joints are the pivoting points where two bones meet, allowing for controlled movement in multiple planes. They consist of:

**Cartilage** - This smooth, elastic tissue coats the ends of bones, enabling them to glide effortlessly over each other with minimal friction. It acts like a cushion, distributing forces and protecting bone.

**Synovial Membrane** - This membrane lines the joint capsule and continuously secretes synovial fluid to lubricate and nourish the cartilage.

**Ligaments** - These fibrous bands of connective tissue stabilize joints by attaching bone to bone, preventing dislocation or excessive movement.

**Tendons** - These cord-like tissues anchor muscle to bone, enabling us to flex and extend our limbs through contraction.

**Bursa** - These small fluid sacs further reduce friction at movement points by creating a gliding surface.

For animal companions to thrive, every component of these intricate joint systems must remain healthy and balanced. When blood flow decreases or inflammatory processes elevate, the tissues can break down faster than the body can repair them. This leads to:

- **Cartilage degeneration** - As cartilage cells deteriorate, bones begin grinding directly together, creating pain, instability and decreased mobility.

- **Joint stiffness** - Decreased synovial fluid production reduces lubrication, causing stiff, painful movements. Activities become difficult.

- **Muscle/Tendon strain** - As pets compensate for painful joints, surrounding muscles and tendons take on excess strain, risking injury.

- **Bone/Tendon spur formations** - The body tries to stabilize deteriorating joints by growing excess bone and fibrotic tissues, which pinch nerves and restrict mobility.

In short, impaired joint health creates a cascade of dysfunction and pain that dramatically compromises a pet's freedom of movement. The resulting inactivity in turn fuels more degeneration, creating a vicious cycle.

Luckily, strategic herbal support comes to the rescue by tackling inflammation, nourishing tissues, and optimizing the entire joint environment. With the right protocol, many pets experience restored mobility and vigor.

**Turmeric:** The Golden Joint Protector
No herbal joint protocol is complete without this Indian spice revered in Ayurveda. Turmeric offers multifaceted support:

**Anti-Inflammatory** - Curcuminoids (notably curcumin) in turmeric are potent anti-inflammatories that work by interrupting inflammatory pathways at the molecular level. This provides relief from swollen, tender joints.

**Analgesic** - Turmeric's pain-relieving effects come from its ability to modulate neurotransmitters involved in pain perception and reduce oxidizing agents that excite pain receptors.

**Antioxidant** - Curcuminoids also act as powerful antioxidants, scavenging free radicals that cause cartilage breakdown. This protects existing joint tissues.

**Regenerative** - Early evidence suggests curcumin primes stem cells involved in cartilage repair while tempering enzymes that deteriorate cartilage.

Contraindications are few, but turmeric can potentially interact with certain medications by increasing bioavailability. It's also recommended to take a break from therapeutic doses periodically.

**Boswellia:** Ancient Herb for Modern Relief Valued in Ayurvedic medicine for millennia, boswellia (also called frankincense) is still considered one of the most versatile botanicals for joint care today:

**Anti-Arthritic** - Boswellic acids reduce inflammation in joints by blocking leukotrienes, prostaglandins and pro-inflammatory enzymes like 5-LOX. Many find boswellia as effective as NSAIDs.

Pain Relief - In addition to quelling inflammation, boswellia prevents the autoimmune reactions that can make joints hypersensitive to pain signals in conditions like rheumatoid arthritis.

Joint Restoration - Studies link boswellia to increases in glycosaminoglycan molecules, which are vital components of cartilage and synovial fluid.

**Cellular Protection** - Antioxidants like terpenoids quench free radicals before they can inflict oxidative damage on joint tissues and cell structures.

**Ginger:** Warming Relief for Achy Joints

With a long culinary history dating back over 5,000 years, ginger's benefits for joint mobility are no joke:

**Potent Anti-Inflammatory** - Gingerol compounds work similarly to COX-2 inhibitors by blocking pro-inflammatory pathways and mediators like interleukin-6.

**Joint Lubrication** - Ginger facilitates smoother synovial fluid production, preventing scar tissue buildup and preserving mobility.

**Circulatory Stimulant** - By increasing oxygenated blood flow to joint areas, ginger speeds delivery of nutrients while flushing inflammatory debris.

**Warming Muscle Relaxant** - The zingy, warming qualities in ginger support healthy muscle function around affected joints while providing soothing pain relief.

Precautions include using small doses for acid reflux sufferers or animals prone to seizures. Monitoring for stomach upset is also wise during initial administration.

Using Herbs in a Joint Support Protocol
There's no one-size-fits-all approach to supporting joint health herbally, as each animal's condition and needs will vary. However, some common protocols tend to work well:

## Foundational Supplement

For general maintenance of healthy joints, start with a base supplement containing turmeric and , formulated for your pet's species and size. This provides daily anti-inflammatory support.

## Acute Flare-Ups

Add ginger and willow bark (a natural source of salicin, similar to aspirin) to the base supplement during acute arthritic flare-ups or injuries to manage pain and swelling.

## Chondroprotection

To support cartilage repair and nutrient delivery, glucosamine, chondroitin, and hyaluronic acid can be added to the base supplement long-term. MSM also aids collagen production.

## Mobility Support

Herbal ingredients like yucca, ashwagandha, and omega-3s can be rotated in to specifically target muscle strength, flexibility, and joint lubrication depending on needs.

## Targeted Topicals

Ointments, salves, and liniments made with capsaicin, peppermint, camphor, menthol, and other botanicals can be massaged into specific joint areas for temporary localized relief.

## Long-Term Restoration

For chronic degenerative conditions, consistent use of the full protocol over 6-12 weeks is usually required to experience maximum benefits as tissues rebuild resiliency.

Always purchase joint supplements from reputable suppliers dealing with certified, high-quality ingredients. Products should clearly display analysis and dosages. Consulting your veterinarian before starting a new regimen is highly recommended as well.

## Combining Modalities for Synergistic Effects

While herbal support is extremely effective, results are often amplified when integrating holistic therapies, particularly for more advanced joint issues:

**Acupuncture** - This ancient practice stimulates strategic pressure points to increase circulation, relieve pain/spasms and rebalance energy pathways around affected joints.

**Chiropractic** - Gentle adjustments relieve subluxations, improving mobility and reducing compensatory strains that exacerbate joint problems.

**Cold Laser Therapy** - Low-level lasers penetrate joint tissues to increase cellular regeneration rates and reduce oxidative damage.

**Massage Therapy** - Strategic massage boosts circulation and restores range of motion in stiff joints while also supporting muscle rehabilitation.

**Physiotherapy** - Stretching and controlled exercises rebuild strength, lubrication and proprioception around joints to restore function.

When combined with phytonutrient support from medicinal plants, these modalities work synergistically to target joint rehabilitation from multiple angles. The key lies in finding your pet's ideal whole-body approach under the guidance of your integrative veterinarian.

One often-overlooked component is managing appropriate weight to avoid excess loading on joint surfaces. Diet and exercise plans tailored to your pet's needs help prevent further degeneration.

## External Support Methods

In addition to oral supplementation and complementary therapies, there are some wonderful topical applications of herbs that enhance relief and rehabilitation:

## Liniments

Applied to specific joint areas, liniments create a warming or cooling sensation that improves circulation while providing temporary localized pain relief. Many contain cayenne, menthol or hemp extracts.

## Salves

Thicker salve preparations deliver anti-inflammatory herbs like , willow bark and St. John's wort directly to affected tissues through absorption. Wax-based bases allow herbs to penetrate deeply.

## Sitz Baths

For hip, knee or other joint areas in the pelvic region, sitz baths let pets soak in warm liquid infused with relaxing herbs like chamomile, calendula or epsom salts.

## Compresses

Using warm or cool herbal tea concentrates like turmeric ginger or comfrey, compresses applied to painful arthritic areas assist healing by enhancing circulation to targeted regions.

## Exercise and Massage Techniques

While medication and passive therapies certainly have their place, actively engaging your pet's body through movement is crucial for preserving joint health long-term. Being sedentary causes muscles to atrophy and joints to seize up, perpetuating disability. Appropriate exercise, when combined with herbal support, massage and other rehab methods, offers numerous benefits:

**Range of Motion** - Controlled joint flexion, extension and rotation exercises pump healing nutrients into joint spaces while preventing scar tissue buildup.

**Muscle Strengthening** - Building supportive muscle stabilizes joints, prevents dislocations, and takes stress off tendons and ligaments to ease arthritic pain.

**Weight Management** - Reducing excess adipose tissue diminishes the constant gravitational load being placed on already compromised joints.

**Increased Circulation** - Pumping blood flow brings rejuvenating oxygen and nutrients while flushing out inflammatory by-products and metabolic wastes.

**Stress Relief** - Endorphins released through movement help regulate pain signals, while the mental enrichment combats anxiety, depression and obsessive behaviors.

Patience and consistency when reintroducing activity is key. Start slowly, use treats/rewards, and integrate herbal supplements to assist comfort levels. In time, your pet can regain their puppy/kitten energy levels!

## Implementing Basic Rehabilitation Routines

So what does a basic home rehab program look like? Here are some veterinarian-approved methods to consider:

**Warm-Up** - Start each session with gentle 360° joint rotations plus slow, easy walks to warm up the tissues and increase blood flow. Build time gradually.

**Controlled Range of Motion** - With your pet in a standing or sternal position, support and guide joints through their full, pain-free motions with your hands.

**Weight Shifting** - Encourage shifting weight back and forth, side to side to build strength/stability through gentle resistance. Go slow. Reward frequently.

**Balance Work** - Having pets walk over/around raised platforms or balance cushions engages stabilizing muscles while increasing proprioception.

**Stretching** - Target the major muscle groups around affected joints by holding supported stretches 5-15 seconds. Never force painful positions.

**Massage** - Using your hands or tools like therapy balls, knead muscles and apply compression around joints to release tension and adhesions.

**Cold/Heat Therapy** - Ice packs post-exercise reduce inflammation. Heat wraps pre-exercise boost circulation and joint fluid production.

**Low-Impact Exercise** - Walking, swimming or using underweight treadmills offers aerobic conditioning without excess impact on healing joints.

Remember to make rehab routines engaging and reward-based. With diligent consistency, most pets begin showing marked progress in mobility within 4-8 weeks when combining herbal and manual therapies. Finding an animal rehab specialist in your area can accelerate recovery even more through customized care.

## The Power of Pet Massage

Of all the hands-on techniques for supporting joint health, therapeutic massage may be my personal favorite. This dynamic modality truly melds the rehabilitative with the nurturing, delivering benefits on both physical and emotional planes. Let's explore how regular massages nurture healthier joints while deepening the human-animal bond:

**Releases Muscle Tension** - Working out knots, adhesions and spasms in muscles that attach around joints creates more freedom for movement with less compensatory strain.

**Improves Circulation** - Strategic compressions along muscle beds pump fresh, oxygenated blood into the area while clearing out inflammatory byproducts and lactic acid buildup.

**Stimulates Proprioception** - Applying traction and resistance encourages pets to engage stabilizing muscles, rekindling awareness of where their body is in space.

**Provides Pain Relief** - Releasing serotonin, endorphins and other "feel good" hormones naturally dampens pain transmission while physically loosening stiff areas.

**Reduces Stress/Anxiety** - Rhythmic massage strokes induce a calm, meditative state that lowers levels of stress hormones like cortisol implicated in inflammatory responses.

**Enhances Mobility/Flexibility** - With relaxed musculature cleared of tension, the full, limber range of joint motion can be restored during and after a massage.

Introduces TLC - The one-on-one contact and devoted touch during a massage strengthens the human-animal bond immensely, conveying love and comfort.

Following your veterinarian's guidance, you can easily incorporate joint-friendly massage into your pet's daily routine. Focus on broad, firm strokes around the hips, shoulders, spine and limb muscles - but always check for tender areas first. Apply medicated ointments or liniments before and after massages to boost relief and absorption. For a real treat, try warm herbal compresses too!

Supplementing With Complementary Care

As you've undoubtedly gathered by now, herbs rarely operate optimally in isolation - they achieve their full rehabilitative power when synergized with other modalities in a multifaceted, whole-body approach. Here's a quick recap of some standout integrative therapies that pair beautifully with herbal joint care:

**Acupuncture** - By removing blockages and rebalancing energy pathways involved with circulation and inflammation, acupuncture enhances herbal benefits.

**Chiropractic** - Realigning subluxations facilitates better herbal delivery to compromised joint areas while relieving compensatory strains.

**Physical Rehabilitation** - Exercises are potentiated when preceded by herbal anti-inflammatories. Herbs also speed tissue recovery after rehab sessions.

**Low-Level Laser** - Used adjunctly, laser treatments increase herbal constituents' cellular bioavailability for faster regenerative results.

**Weight Management** - Herbally-supported diets ease systemic inflammation that exacerbates excess weight gain and joint deterioration.

Finding an integrative veterinarian well-versed in complementary modalities is key to orchestrating a cohesive game plan. Monitor your pet's progress continually and make adjustments to their tailored protocol over time. With patience and consistency, a multimodal approach can make all the difference in preserving quality of life through the golden years!

I hope this chapter has illuminated the pivotal roles botanicals like turmeric, and ginger can play in maintaining mobility and joint comfort as our animal friends age. Backed by the latest research yet rooted in traditions stretching back centuries, these herbs offer a gentle, restorative means of nurturing resilience in the pivots that allow our companions to thrive.

Yet herbs are truly at their best when unified with other modalities like massage, rehabilitation, acupuncture and more under the guidance of an integrative veterinarian. Patience and consistency with a multimodal protocol rewards us by keeping our treasured companions nimble, active and gleefully engaged with life well into their twilight years.

So stay the course, shower your pet with TLC through massage and quality care, and look forward to enjoying their playful, spirited presence for as long as possible. When it comes to preserving the joy of unfettered mobility, nature's bounty has your back!

# Chapter 4

# Anxiety and Stress Relief

In an increasingly frenetic world filled with loud noises, unpredictable schedules, and a million tiny triggers, it's no wonder so many of our beloved animal companions struggle with anxiety and stress. Pent-up nervous energy frequently manifests in disruptive behaviors like incessant barking, destructive chewing, inappropriate elimination, obsessive grooming, and even self-mutilation. More than just inconvenient, chronic stress unleashes cascades of physiological consequences that erode our pets' quality of life.

While conventional treatments like prescription anti-anxiety medications certainly provide relief for severe cases, many caring pet parents understandably wish to first explore gentler, more natural solutions. Luckily, Mother Nature has gifted us with a soothing botanical pharmacy stocked with mild, non-habit-forming calmatives and mood-regulators. This chapter will empower you to craft herbal protocols for reigning in anxiety while nurturing emotional well-being holistically.

In the following pages, we'll spotlight key herbs like chamomile, valerian, and lemon balm that relieve tension through gentle sedation. You'll learn soothing essential oil combinations ideal for diffusing or massage. We'll also discuss proactive strategies like environmental enrichment, exercise routines, and nutritional adjustments to address anxiety's underlying root causes. By blending herbal remedies, lifestyle modifications, and some good old-fashioned TLC, you can help restore your pet's confidence and centered state of mind.

## The Physiological Impacts of Chronic Stress

Before we dive into botanical solutions, it's helpful to first understand exactly how detrimental chronic anxiety can be on the body, mind and spirit. The effects of unresolved stress extend far beyond behavioral disruptions:

**Immune Suppression** - Continually elevated levels of stress hormones like cortisol suppress normal immune function, leaving pets vulnerable to infections and diseases.

**Inflammation Response** - Stress triggers a chain reaction of inflammatory processes that when persistent, can damage organs, joints, and neurological pathways.

**Gastrointestinal Distress** - Both physical and psychological stressors immediately disrupt gut health, causing stomach upset, diarrhea, decreased nutrient absorption, and more.

**Accelerated Aging** - Increased oxidative strain from stress takes a toll on cells and

DNA, creating accelerated "wear and tear" on organs and longevity.

**Hormone Imbalance** - Abnormal production of neurotransmitters, sexual hormones and thyroid hormones lead to metabolic issues, emotional imbalance, and reproductive problems.

**Weight Fluctuations** - Stress impacts appetite hormones, either triggering irrational urges to overeat and gain weight or reducing hunger entirely leading to muscle wasting.

**Cardiovascular Impacts** - Persistent anxiety and panic elevate blood pressure, heart rate, and stroke risk while accelerating the progression of coronary disease.

**Behavioral Changes** - Beyond outright anxiety, stressed pets often exhibit problematic behaviors stemming from excess energy, irritability, insecurity, and lack of focus.

**Quality of Life** - When anxiety and nerves become an everyday experience, the constant hyper-vigilance and unease severely diminishes joy, playfulness, and overall vitality.

As you can see, chronic stress wreaks havoc across all physiological systems, creating acute and chronic conditions with long-term repercussions. While herbal calmatives provide valuable relief, a more holistic, proactive approach is required to truly curb anxiety at its neurochemical roots.

**Chamomile:** Harbinger of Inner Peace
Let's begin our botanical journey into anxiolytic (anti-anxiety) herbs with a calming superstar already growing in many backyards:

Chamomile has been revered as a mild sedative across cultures for thousands of years. This gentle daisy delivers soothing benefits through:

**Glycine Complex** - Glycine, an inhibitory amino acid, binds receptors in the brain to decrease neurological activity, inducing calm. Other glycine complex compounds magnify this effect.

**Flavonoid Antioxidants** - Polyphenols like apigenin exert adaptogenic properties, helping regulate mood and protect neurons from stress-induced damage over time.

**Anti-Inflammatory Actions** - The azulene compounds in chamomile temper inflammation that exacerbates anxiety and associated gastrointestinal symptoms like nausea or diarrhea.

**Muscle Relaxant Properties** - The sedative effects help melt away physical tension, paving the way for deep, restorative rest to combat depleted energy levels.

Chamomile is gentle enough for pets of all ages, from puppies and kittens up to senior animals. Studies show it can safely be given daily over extended periods unlike anti-anxiety medications. It's especially useful for situational stressors like thunderstorms or travel, but offers lasting ease when used as part of an overall lifestyle regimen.

**Valerian Root:** Plant-Based Peaceful Slumber

In the world of calming herbs, valerian root stands as one of the most clinically researched and widely trusted sedatives for overcoming insomnia. Its anti-anxiety powers make it equally valuable for managing pet stress:

**GABA/Serotonin Modulation** - Valerian acts on GABA receptors, exerting a soothing effect on the central nervous system while helping produce calming serotonin.

**Muscle Relaxation** - It contains compounds called valepotriates, which act similarly to benzodiazepines like Valium™, helping unwind physical and mental tension before bedtime.

**Improved Sleep Cycles** - Modulation of GABA also regulates sleep/wake cycles and circadian rhythms to combat insomnia and promote restorative rest.

**Possible Anti-Depressant Effects** - By influencing serotonin and melatonin, valerian may provide mood elevation and combat the fatigue associated with anxiety.

The roots possess a rather distinct earthy, pungent scent which animals sometimes find unappealing at first. We'll discuss masking techniques when making treats shortly! Valerian should not be given long-term, as receptor downregulation requires periodic breaks. But for situational or short bursts of nervousness, valerian provides gentle sedation.

**Passionflower:** Cosmic Calm at the Interface

Drawing on traditions from both Native American and European herbalism, the passion flower plant lends its mild tranquilizing properties:

**Anti-Anxiety Alkaloids** - harmala alkaloids like harman increase GABA receptor sensitivity while modulating serotonin and dopamine pathways in the brain. The result is a sense of calmness.

**Antioxidant/Anti-Inflammatory-** Flavonoids like apigenin and chrysin help reverse oxidative stress and inflammation associated with anxiety states, fatigue and malaise.

**Muscle Relaxant/Sleep Aid** - Through sedative benzoflavone compounds, passionflower extracts may improve sleep quality and quantity by unwinding physical tension.

**Analgesic Properties** - The pain-relieving effects of passionflower can combat aches and stress-induced hyperalgesia (increased pain sensitivity).

**Passionflower delivers results fast -** often within 30 minutes of administration. Yet it tends to feel less overtly sedating than valerian with no morning "hangover" effect for anxiety sufferers. It's gentle enough for daily use across all life stages.

When combined, these "big three" **anti-anxiety herbs - chamomile, valerian, and passionflower** - create powerful synergies for safe, effective, multi-layered relief. But they're just the beginning! Let's look at more versatile herbal allies and some unique applications.

## Calming Essential Oil Blends

For calming particularly hyper pets prone to excess barking, pacing, scratching or other anxious behaviors, blends of essential oils provide "on the spot" relief. Simply diffusing soothing aromas or misting onto bedding offers passive chill-out power:

**Grounding Oils:**
- Vetiver, clary sage, sandalwood, frankincense, cedarwood

**Relaxing Florals:**
- Lavender, chamomile, rose, ylang-ylang, jasmine, neroli

**Fruity/Minty Oils:**

- Sweet orange, bergamot, grapefruit, lemon, peppermint

**Classic Calming Blend Recipe:**

4 drops bergamot

3 drops lavender

2 drops chamomile roman

2 drops clary sage

1 drop sandalwood

Diffuse up to 1 hour, reapplying as needed. Excellent for storms!

Always use only pure, high-quality essential oils formulated for pets. The potent plant compounds work quickly to trigger the parasympathetic "rest and digest" response through the olfactory system. You'll notice pets start taking deep calming breaths when properly dosed.

My favorite "active" application involves whipping up a soothing body butter for anxiety-relieving pet massages:

Super-Calm Massage Butter
1/4 cup organic shea butter
1/4 cup coconut oil (solid but soft)
10 drops lavender essential oil
6 drops bergamot essential oil
5 drops sweet orange or neroli essential oil

Mash all ingredients together well. Scoop out and melt a small amount into your hands, then gently massage into your pet's neck, ears, chest, and spine as they relax into the soothing strokes. Inhaling those botanical aromas while releasing muscular tension creates pure bliss!

The key when using essential oil treatments? Always buy high-quality oils from reputable sources, follow dilution guidelines closely, and first introduce aromas slowly to avoid potential sensitivities. A little patience and these subtle scents take the edge off!

## Soothing Nervine Herbs for Deep Calm

In the Western medicinal tradition, herbs traditionally used for supporting nervous system health are classified as "nervines" - a highly valuable category. Some of these herbal allies soothe the psyche through relaxation, while others actively nourish, protect and restore frayed nerves over time. Together, they form synergistic teams combating anxiety from multiple fronts.

On the instantaneous nervine sedative front, we find calming friends like:

Lemon Balm - Rosmarinic acid helps uplift the mood while mildly quieting the mind. Excellent for ADHD anxiety, as the focusing effects balance sedation.

Skullcap - The flavonoids in skullcap ease nervous overexcitability, moodiness, muscle spasms, and insomnia without impairing energy or mental clarity. Good for hyperarousal.

**Motherwort** - An age-old heart/uterus tonic used to relieve anxiety-induced palpitations, hot flashes, and hormonal mood swings. Eases stress while cooling inflammation.

**Kava Kava** - This South Pacific root profoundly eases muscular tension and fatigue while promoting mental tranquility. Use with extreme caution and monitor for liver effects.

Nervine tonics provide more rehabilitative, longer-term support by restoring optimal nervous system function. Top allies include:

**Oat Seed** - A classic restorative for frazzled, depleted nerves after periods of overexertion or fright. Returns balance over time while rejuvenating mental focus.

**Milky Oats** - Similar to their mature counterparts, milky oat tops and seeds have a slightly more sedative influence perfect for anxiety, addictions and exhaustion.

**Ashwagandha** - This adaptogenic "Indian ginseng" boosts neurotransmitters like GABA, while defending the brain/nerves against oxidative stresses that exacerbate anxiety.

**Eleuthero Root** - Another adaptogen, but more stimulating than ashwagandha - eleuthero enhances resilience to stressors and increases endurance over time.

**St. John's Wort** - The hypericin compounds have strong anti-anxiety and antidepressant properties by optimizing serotonin and GABA pathways while offering neuroprotection.

While less well-known, these versatile tonics make wonderful additions to other calming herbs and lifestyle adjustments for managing anxiety from all angles. Rotating them seasonally can help avoid plateaus and sustain adaptability.

## Diet: Balancing Nutrients for Optimal Brain Health

Did you know the food pets eat provides the nutritional backbone to either exacerbate or alleviate anxiety? Whole, high-quality fresh foods supply not just energy, but the building blocks for producing neurotransmitters involved in emotional regulation like serotonin, dopamine, GABA and melatonin. When dietary intake becomes imbalanced, it can directly impact mood, impulse control and stress resilience.

Here are some key nutrient groups and food sources to focus on when crafting an anti-anxiety diet:

**Omega-3 Fatty Acids** - From fatty fish, flax/chia seeds, and marine algae, these essential fats form the basic membrane architecture for neuronal communication. They optimize serotonin levels.

**Tryptophan** - Found in turkey, oats, bananas, and milk, tryptophan converts into serotonin and melatonin, master regulators of circadian rhythms, stress responses and positive mood.

**B Vitamins** - These water-soluble vitamins, especially B1, B5, B6, B9 and B12 found in liver, greens, and nutritional yeast facilitate neurotransmitter synthesis while protecting nerve fibers.

**Magnesium** - Crucial for GABA receptor binding and moderating glutamate (an excitatory neurotransmitter), magnesium from seeds/nuts calms the nervous system.

**Anti-Inflammatory Foods** - Chronic inflammation exacerbates anxiety, so focus on antioxidant-packed foods like turmeric, tart cherries, green tea, and colorful produce.

**Low-Glycemic Carbs** - Whole grains, beans, lentils and sweet potatoes sustain steady blood sugar to prevent mood/energy crashes linked to anxiety and hyperactivity.

**Hydrating Foods** - Proper water balance from moisture-rich veggies, broths, and unsweetened juices optimizes neurotransmitter flow and detoxification.

Limiting-hyperstimulation, highly-processed foods devoid of nutritive value while emphasizing whole-food sources gives nature's anxiety-relieving compounds the best chance to work. Pets feel more grounded both physically and mentally.

You can easily supplement a fresh diet by incorporating nervine herbs into home-cooked meals, treats, and hydrating teas - let's take a look at some favorite recipes using botanical sedatives and tonics!

## Herbal Remedy Blends and Concoctions

While isolated herbs certainly shine, they often work better together synergistically in formulations targeting certain effects. Here are some classic anti-anxiety/calming herbal remedy blends incorporating various sedative and tonic herbs:

Happy Camper Tea

- Ingredients: Chamomile, lemon balm, oatstraw

- Effects: Calms jitters, soothes frayed nerves, gently sedates

- Use: Cool completely and serve as the base for hydrating liquid meals, cocktails, or just offer plain as a treat during stressful times.

Serenity Now Tincture

- Ingredients: Motherwort, linden flower, skullcap, valerian root

- Effects: Eases anxieties, tension headaches, hormonal mood swings, insomnia

- Use: Administer standard dropper doses by mouth or dilute and mist onto bedding or onto the body.

Mel's Herbal Chill Pills

- Ingredients: Passionflower, chamomile, ginger, honey

- Effects: Fast-acting mild sedative for calming anxiety, car ride nerves, or hyperactivity

- Use: Roll into little balls and give 30-60 minutes prior to stressful events or at bedtime.

Brain Reboot Elixir

- Ingredients: Milky oats, ashwagandha, St. John's wort, eleuthero

- Effects: Deeply nourishing for depleted, overstimulated nervous systems.

- Use: Add tinctured herbs to bone broth or herbal tea and sip daily to restore balance over time.

Aroma-Mutt-Apy Spritz

- Ingredients: Vodka or witch hazel, plus 5-7 calming essential oils of choice

- Effects: Instantly soothing for high-anxiety situations or travel

- Use: Mist environment, bedding or pet's body when needed to trigger parasympathetic "chill" mode.

The true beauty of herbal remedies lies in how infinitely customizable they are! Feel free to adapt these blends or craft new ones to suit your pet's specific needs and responsiveness. Keeping a journal can help track what works.

Exercise, Enrichment and Other De-Stressing Techniques

While herbal calmatives and dietary support provide important neurochemical relief for anxious pets, we'd be remiss to ignore behavioral modification and lifestyle enrichment strategies. Meeting your animal companion's innate needs for daily enrichment, exercise, confident handling and positive routines actually targets anxiety's root causes.

Environmental Enrichment

Contrary to popular belief, leaving pets alone for hours in barren, cramped environments often exacerbates anxiety and related problematic behaviors. Basic enrichment activities keep minds and bodies engaged:

- Food Puzzle Toys - Having to work and problem-solve by manipulating objects provides the mental stimulation and sense of control animals crave.

- Scent Enrichment - Introducing novel smells like herbs, spices or pheremonally-enriched toys engages their keen olfactory senses.

- Rotated Toys - Providing a rotation of different toys, fabrics and exploratory items prevents boredom while reinforcing curiosity.

- Outdoor Access - Supervised time outdoors enables natural behaviors like digging, exploring new smells, and experiencing varied sensations.

- Clicker Training - Positive reinforcement clicker training builds confidence while alleviating pent-up energy through mental exercises.

Frequent rotation and switching up enrichment items creates that all-important novelty and unpredictability mammals need to feel enriched.

Exercise and Playtime
Physical activity provides an invaluable outlet for releasing pent-up energy, restlessness and anxiety through healthy avenues. Engage your pet daily through:

- Walks/Hikes - The basic act of smelling new scents while moving in nature has remarkably calming effects on the canine/feline psyche.

- Games - Chase, fetch, and social play help reinforce hierarchical roles, build confidence, and forge trust between pet and owner.

- Agility/Tricks - Setting achievable challenges accesses their natural athleticism and problem-solving drive, inspiring feelings of capability.

- Swimming - Working different muscle groups through low-impact exercises like swimming can be incredibly therapeutic.

- Pet Massage - Post-activity massages cement bonding while relieving any muscular tension or residual cortisol release.

Aerobic activity releases mood-regulating endorphins while strengthening the cardiovascular system for oxygenated calm focus. Pair it with enrichment for maximal stress relief!

Routine and Predictability
While novelty satisfies innate curiosities, pets also crave reliable routines that create feelings of safety and control over their environment. Predictable patterns like:

- Scheduled Feedings - Following a consistent meal timing and preparation routine prevents obsessive behaviors around food.

- Potty Outings - Taking them out regularly averts indoor accidents while reinforcing good bathroom habits alleviates stress.

- Wake/Sleep Cycles - Sticking to normal activity and winding down schedules regulates circadian rhythms for adequate rest.

- Exposure Practice - Gradually introducing potentially triggering stimuli in controlled doses helps desensitize fears.

- Obedience Training - Basic commands like "stay" foster impulse control while reinforcing feelings of confidence and security.

While variety is the spice of life, overarching familiarity creates anchors of reassurance that prevent feeling overwhelmed by stimuli. Merging routine with appropriate enrichment hits the sweet spot!

Calming Tools and Modifications
Sometimes pets need a little extra assistance managing anxieties, especially during triggering events. Integrate calming tools and modifications like:

- Pheromones - Synthetic analogs of natural pheromones found effective for reducing stress levels and related behaviors.

- Body Wraps - Gentle pressure from snug-fitting wraps, capes or shirts can have a grounding, swaddling effect for some pets.

- White Noise - Soothing ambient sounds like air diffusers or recorded bathroom fan noises help mask startling external triggers.

- Calming Caps/Hoods - These soft fabric accessories create a slight visual "blinding" that dampens sensory overload for storm or noise phobias.

- Counter Surfing - Temporarily restricting access to certain areas or perches where anxious behaviors manifest.

- Herbal Tinctures - Fast-acting liquid herbal extracts quickly elicit the parasympathetic "rest and digest" response when needed.

The key lies in figuring out each individual pet's needs and introducing supportive tools through positive reinforcement to avoid creating aversions or new anxieties.

Combining these behavioral, environmental, and lifestyle techniques with the internal nutritional and herbal support we've discussed creates a powerful 360° approach to combating anxiety at every level. With commitment and patience, even the most nervous pets can regain calmness!

# Chapter 5

# Digestive Health and Detoxification for Pets

## Introduction

As a veterinarian, one of the most common concerns I encounter among pet owners is the well-being of their furry companions' digestive systems. A healthy digestive tract is the foundation for overall vitality, energy, and longevity in our beloved pets. In this chapter, we'll embark on an exploration of digestive health and detoxification specifically tailored for our four-legged friends.

Throughout our journey, we'll delve into the world of demulcents, bitters, probiotics, and gut-healthy foods, uncovering their unique benefits and how they can contribute to optimal digestive function in our canine and feline companions. Whether your pet is dealing with occasional discomfort or you're seeking to enhance their body's natural detoxification processes, this chapter promises to provide you with valuable insights and practical solutions.

So, let's embark on this exploration together, embracing the wisdom of nature and empowering ourselves with the knowledge to cultivate a thriving digestive system for our beloved pets – the foundation of vibrant health and happiness.

Demulcents: Soothing the Sensitive Digestive Tracts of Pets

As any pet owner knows, our furry companions can be susceptible to digestive upsets, ranging from occasional discomfort to more persistent issues. In these delicate situations, the gentle and soothing properties of demulcents can be a true blessing for our pets' sensitive digestive tracts.

One of the most revered demulcents in the world of pet health is slippery elm. Derived from the inner bark of the Ulmus tree, slippery elm boasts a rich history of use by indigenous communities for various ailments, particularly those related to the gastrointestinal tract. Its unique composition, rich in mucilage, a soothing and lubricating substance, allows it to form a protective barrier along the digestive tract, shielding it from irritation and inflammation.

But slippery elm's benefits extend far beyond its soothing properties. This remarkable plant possesses antioxidant and anti-inflammatory compounds that can help mitigate the effects of oxidative stress and reduce inflammation, two key contributors to digestive discomfort in pets. Additionally, its prebiotic properties nourish the beneficial bacteria that reside in our pets' gut, promoting a healthy and balanced microbiome.

Incorporating slippery elm into your pet's diet can be as simple as mixing it into their food or offering it as a soothing treat. Its gentle, slightly sweet taste and versatility make it a delightful addition to any pet wellness regimen. However, as with any supplement, it's essential to consult with your veterinarian to determine the appropriate dosage and ensure it's safe for your pet's specific needs.

Bitters: Awakening the Digestive Fire in Pets

While demulcents soothe and protect, bitters awaken and stimulate the digestive process in our beloved pets, igniting a symphony of enzymatic activity and bile flow. Among the most revered bitters in the natural world for pet health is the humble yet powerful dandelion.

Often overlooked as a mere weed, the dandelion harbors a treasure trove of digestive benefits for our furry friends. Its roots, leaves, and flowers are rich in bitter compounds, including sesquiterpene lactones and phenolic acids, which act as natural digestive tonics. When these compounds interact with the taste receptors on our pets' tongues, they trigger a cascade of physiological responses, including increased salivation, gastric acid secretion, and bile production – all essential components of optimal digestion.

But dandelion's virtues extend far beyond its bitterness. This resilient plant is a potent detoxifier, supporting the liver's natural ability to eliminate toxins and metabolic waste products in our pets. Its diuretic properties further aid in the removal of harmful substances from the body, promoting a gentle yet effective cleansing process.

Incorporating dandelion into your pet's diet can be as simple as adding its leaves to their meals or offering them as a healthy treat. For a more concentrated dose of its bitterness, consider brewing a warm cup of dandelion root tea and adding a small amount to their water bowl, allowing the earthy, slightly bitter flavor to awaken their digestive fire.

## Probiotics and Gut-Healthy Foods: Cultivating a Thriving Microbiome in Pets

Within the intricate ecosystem of our pets' digestive tracts resides a vast and diverse community of microscopic inhabitants – the gut microbiome. This intricate web of bacteria, archaea, fungi, and viruses plays a crucial role in our pets' overall health, influencing everything from digestion and nutrient absorption to immune function and even their mental well-being.

To nurture and support this delicate microbial balance, we must embrace the power of probiotics and gut-healthy foods.

Probiotics, often referred to as "friendly bacteria," are living microorganisms that, when consumed in adequate amounts, confer a host of health benefits to their host – our beloved pets.

One of the most widely recognized and studied probiotics for pets is the Lactobacillus family, which includes strains like Lactobacillus acidophilus, Lactobacillus , and Lactobacillus plantarum. These beneficial bacteria not only aid in digestion and nutrient absorption but also play a crucial role in maintaining a healthy gut barrier in our pets, preventing the influx of harmful substances and pathogens.

However, probiotics alone are not enough to sustain a thriving microbiome in our furry companions. We must also nourish these vital allies with a diverse array of gut-healthy foods rich in prebiotics – the "food" that fuels the growth and activity of our pets' beneficial gut inhabitants.

Fermented foods, such as kefir or goat's milk yogurt, can be excellent sources of both probiotics and prebiotics for our pets, providing a synergistic blend of live cultures and fiber to support a balanced gut ecosystem. Additionally, incorporating fiber-rich fruits and vegetables like pumpkin, sweet potatoes, and green beans into your pet's diet ensures a steady supply of prebiotic fuel, fostering a diverse and resilient microbiome.

By embracing probiotics and gut-healthy foods, we cultivate an environment that supports optimal digestive function, nutrient absorption, and overall well-being in our pets – a true testament to the interconnectedness of their bodies and the microscopic world within.

## Conclusion

As we conclude our exploration of digestive health and detoxification for our beloved pets, we are reminded of the profound wisdom embodied by nature's remedies. From the soothing embrace of demulcents like slippery elm to the awakening power of bitters like dandelion, and the nurturing of a thriving gut microbiome through probiotics and gut-healthy foods, we have uncovered a wealth of knowledge that can guide us towards vibrant digestive health for our furry companions.

Remember, our pets' digestive systems are the gateway to nourishment, the foundation upon which their bodies build and thrive. By embracing these natural allies and integrating them into their daily lives, we can unleash the full potential of their bodies' innate healing and detoxification capabilities.

So, let us embark on this journey of compassionate care and nourishment for our pets, armed with the insights and practical wisdom gained from this chapter. May their digestive fires burn brightly, their gut microbiomes flourish, and their bodies' natural detoxification processes flow with ease, paving the way for radiant health, vitality, and happiness.

As veterinary professionals, it is our duty to continually expand our knowledge and seek out the most effective and gentle approaches to supporting the well-being of our beloved animal companions. By embracing the wisdom of nature and combining it with modern scientific understanding, we can provide our pets with the highest level of care and ensure their journey through life is filled with vibrant health and joy.

# Chapter 6

# Immune System Support for Pets

In the ever-changing landscape of modern life, our beloved pets face a multitude of challenges that can put strain on their immune systems. From environmental toxins and stress to the natural aging process, their bodies are constantly working to maintain a delicate balance and defend against potential threats. It is our responsibility as devoted pet owners to provide them with the tools they need to thrive, and one of the most powerful weapons in their arsenal is a robust and resilient immune system.

Throughout this chapter, we will embark on a journey of discovery, exploring the natural world's bountiful offerings and how they can be harnessed to fortify our furry companions' defenses. We will delve into the realms of herbs like astragalus, echinacea, and elderberry, each with its unique abilities to bolster immunity, and uncover the secrets of preventative care through nutrition, stress management, and routine veterinary visits.

But with great power comes great responsibility, and we must also navigate the delicate terrain of autoimmune conditions, ensuring that our efforts to strengthen the immune system do not inadvertently exacerbate these complex disorders. Fear not, for we shall guide you through this intricate landscape, armed with knowledge and wisdom, so that you can make informed decisions that prioritize the well-being of your cherished companions.

Herbs like astragalus, echinacea, and elderberry are potent allies in boosting the immune system of our beloved pets. These natural remedies, with their unique properties and rich histories, offer a holistic approach to supporting our companions' overall health and vitality. Let's delve deeper into the world of these botanical wonders and explore how we can harness their powers to address various health concerns in our furry friends.

## Astragalus: The Adaptogenic Ally

Astragalus, an unassuming root with a long-standing reputation in traditional Chinese medicine, has gained recognition for its remarkable adaptogenic properties. This means that it helps the body adapt to stress, a common culprit in immune system suppression and various health issues.

One of the primary ways astragalus supports immune function is by modulating the activity of various immune cells, including macrophages, natural killer cells, and T-cells. These cells play crucial roles in identifying and neutralizing potential threats, such as viruses, bacteria, and even cancerous cells. By enhancing their activity, astragalus bolsters our pets' defenses, making them better equipped to ward off infections and other health challenges.

But astragalus's benefits extend far beyond immune support. This versatile herb has been shown to have anti-inflammatory properties, making it a valuable ally in managing conditions like arthritis and joint pain, which are common concerns for many pets, especially as they age.

To incorporate astragalus into your pet's routine, you can consider the following options:

1. **Astragalus Decoction:** Prepare a decoction by simmering the dried root in water for an extended period. Once cooled,

you can mix a small amount of the liquid into your pet's food or water bowl.

2. **Astragalus Powder:** Look for high-quality astragalus powder or capsules, which can be sprinkled over your pet's meals or administered directly (after consulting with your veterinarian for proper dosing).

3. **Astragalus Treats:** Get creative in the kitchen and bake astragalus powder into tasty, homemade treats for your furry friend. This can be a fun and delicious way to introduce this powerful herb into their diet.

**Echinacea:** The Immune System's Champion

Echinacea, with its striking purple petals and hardy demeanor, has long been revered for its immune-boosting properties. This North American native is rich in compounds like alkylamides, polysaccharides, and caffeic acid derivatives, which have been shown to stimulate various aspects of the immune system.

One of echinacea's primary mechanisms of action is its ability to activate macrophages and natural killer cells, two essential components of the innate immune response. These cells act as the body's first line of defense against invading pathogens, engulfing and destroying them before they can cause harm.

Echinacea has also been found to support the production of cytokines, which are signaling molecules that help coordinate the immune system's response. By modulating cytokine levels, echinacea can help maintain a balanced and effective immune response, ensuring that our pets' defenses are primed and ready to combat potential threats.

To incorporate echinacea into your pet's routine, consider the following options:

1. **Echinacea Tincture:** Look for high-quality echinacea tinctures made from fresh or dried plant material. These can be added to your pet's food or water bowl, following the recommended dosage from your veterinarian or a qualified herbalist.

2. **Echinacea Supplements:** Many pet-specific echinacea supplements are available in the form of chews, powders, or capsules. These can be a convenient way to ensure your pet receives a consistent dose of this powerful herb.

3. **Echinacea Tea:** For a more natural approach, you can brew echinacea tea by steeping the dried herb in hot water. Once cooled, you can add a small amount to your pet's water bowl or mix it into their food.

**Elderberry:** The Antioxidant Powerhouse

Elderberry, an unassuming shrub with deep-purple berries, has gained a well-deserved reputation as an immune-boosting superstar. This humble plant is packed with antioxidants, including anthocyanins and flavonoids, which not only support the immune system but also help mitigate the damaging effects of oxidative stress.

Oxidative stress is a major contributing factor to chronic inflammation and various health issues, from arthritis to cancer. By providing a potent source of antioxidants, elderberry helps neutralize harmful free radicals and protect our pets' cells from oxidative damage, thereby supporting overall health and vitality.

But elderberry's benefits don't stop there. Research has shown that this remarkable berry possesses anti-viral properties, making it a valuable ally in supporting respiratory health and combating seasonal illnesses. Its ability to modulate the immune system's response can help prevent overreaction, which is often the cause of severe symptoms during viral infections.

To incorporate elderberry into your pet's routine, consider the following options:

1. **Elderberry Syrup:** Look for high-quality, pet-safe elderberry syrups that you can easily mix into your companion's food or water bowl. These syrups are often combined with other immune-boosting ingredients like honey and ginger for added benefits.

2. **Elderberry Powder or Capsules:** For a more concentrated dose, you can find

elderberry powder or capsules made specifically for pets. These can be sprinkled over their meals or administered directly, following your veterinarian's guidance.

**3. Elderberry Gummies or Treats:** Many pet supplement companies now offer elderberry-infused gummies or treats, making it easy and fun to give your furry friend a daily dose of this powerful antioxidant.

Remember, while these herbs offer remarkable benefits, it's essential to consult with your veterinarian or a qualified herbalist before introducing any new supplement into your pet's routine. They can help ensure proper dosing, identify potential interactions with existing medications, and provide guidance on the most appropriate form and administration method for your pet's specific needs.

By embracing the power of astragalus, echinacea, and elderberry, you're investing in your pet's overall health and well-being, providing them with the natural tools they need to thrive in the face of life's challenges. With a little creativity and guidance, these botanical allies can become a delightful and nourishing addition to your companion's daily routine, fortifying their immune system and supporting their journey towards vibrant health.

## Preventative Care: A Holistic Approach

While herbal remedies can be powerful allies in boosting our pets' immune systems, true resilience lies in a holistic approach that encompasses all aspects of their well-being. Preventative care is the cornerstone of this philosophy, a proactive stance that seeks to fortify our companions' defenses before they are challenged.

At the heart of preventative care lies a nutrient-dense diet, tailored to our pets' unique needs and life stage. A balanced and species-appropriate diet, rich in antioxidants, vitamins, and minerals, provides the building blocks for a robust immune system. From lean proteins and healthy fats to an abundance of fresh fruits and vegetables, every morsel we offer our furry friends contributes to their overall vitality.

But nutrition is just one piece of the puzzle. Stress, that insidious force that can wreak havoc on our pets' mental and physical health, must also be addressed. By creating a calm and enriching environment, filled with opportunities for play, exercise, and mental stimulation, we can help mitigate the negative impacts of stress on their immune function.

Routine veterinary visits are another cornerstone of preventative care. These regular check-ups not only allow for early detection and intervention of potential health issues but also provide valuable opportunities for education and guidance on maintaining optimal immune health.

Autoimmune Considerations: Treading Carefully

While the prospect of boosting our pets' immune systems may seem universally beneficial, there is a delicate balance to be struck when it comes to autoimmune conditions. In these complex disorders, the body's own defense mechanisms mistakenly attack healthy tissues, leading to inflammation and potentially severe complications.

When working with immunomodulators, substances that can either stimulate or suppress the immune system, caution must be exercised in pets with autoimmune disorders. Certain herbs, like echinacea, which are renowned for their immune-boosting properties, may inadvertently exacerbate symptoms in these delicate cases.

It is crucial to consult with a veterinarian who specializes in integrative or holistic medicine when considering the use of immunomodulators in pets with autoimmune conditions. These professionals possess a deep understanding of the intricate interplay between the immune system and these disorders, and can guide you in making informed decisions that prioritize your pet's safety and well-being.

In some cases, gentle immune-modulating herbs like licorice root or reishi mushroom may be recommended, as they can help restore balance and regulate the immune response without overstimulation. Additionally, dietary interventions, stress management techniques, and targeted supplementation may be employed to support immune health while minimizing the risk of flare-ups.

**The Road Ahead:** A Journey of Compassion and Wisdom

As we navigate the intricate landscape of immune system support for our beloved pets, we are reminded of the profound interconnectedness of all aspects of their well-being. From the natural remedies that fortify their defenses to the preventative measures that cultivate resilience, each component plays a vital role in fostering a robust and harmonious immune response.

It is a journey that requires patience, dedication, and a deep respect for the wisdom of nature and modern veterinary science. By embracing a holistic approach and remaining vigilant to the unique needs of our furry companions, we can empower them to thrive, even in the face of life's challenges.

So, let us embark on this path together, armed with knowledge, compassion, and an unwavering commitment to the well-being of our cherished pets. For in their eyes, we see not just companions, but faithful friends and family members whose health and happiness are inextricably intertwined with our own.

# Chapter 7

# Herbal Nutrition and Dietary Supplements - Nature's Bounty for Your Furry (or Feathered) Friend

Have you ever glanced at your pet, luxuriating in a sunbeam, and thought, "There's something missing from their diet?" Perhaps their coat isn't quite as lustrous as it could be, or maybe their energy level seems a touch low. As a veterinarian, I'm here to tell you that nature has provided a treasure trove of options to address these concerns — a world of herbal nutrition and dietary supplements.

Now, before you envision bowls overflowing with strange-looking plants, let me assure you, incorporating herbal powerhouses into your pet's diet can be both simple and incredibly beneficial. This chapter dives deep into the fascinating realm of herbal support for our furry (or feathered) companions. We'll explore the hidden potential of everyday plants like seaweed, nettle, and alfalfa, unraveling the science behind their benefits for our animal friends.

But venturing into the world of supplements requires responsible navigation. We'll delve into crucial guidelines for safe supplementation, taking into account your pet's species, size, and specific needs. It's not a one-size-fits-all approach! Understanding these factors ensures your pet gets the right amount of herbal goodness without any unwanted side effects.

Of course, theory is only half the fun. To get you started on this exciting journey, I'll be sharing some awesomeor wing-tastic!) recipes for incorporating these herbal wonders into your pet's meals. Imagine enticing herbal teas for your cat, soothing broths for your dog, or even nutritious meal toppers that will have your pet begging for more.

By the end of this chapter, you'll be equipped with the knowledge and tools to make informed decisions about incorporating herbal nutrition and dietary supplements into your pet's life. Remember, a healthy pet is a happy pet, and sometimes, a little nudge from nature can make all the difference.

So, buckle up, pet parents! We're about to embark on an enriching exploration of the wonders of herbal support for our cherished companions.

## Unveiling the Power of Plants: A Look at Seaweed, Nettle, and Alfalfa

Mother Nature's medicine cabinet is overflowing with potent plant allies, each boasting unique properties that can benefit our pets' health. Let's delve into three particularly noteworthy examples:

- **Seaweed:** This unassuming aquatic plant is a treasure trove of vitamins and minerals. Packed with vitamins A,

C, and E, seaweed acts as a powerful antioxidant, protecting your pet's cells from damage. It's also a rich source of iodine, essential for proper thyroid function, and can even contribute to a healthy, shiny coat.

However, the true magic lies in the prebiotics found in seaweed. These prebiotics nurture the good bacteria in your pet's gut, promoting healthy digestion and a robust immune system. Think of it as a natural internal fertilizer, ensuring your pet thrives from the inside out.

- **Nettle:** Don't let the name fool you! This common garden weed is a powerhouse of essential vitamins and minerals, including iron, calcium, and magnesium. Nettle leaves are particularly beneficial for pets with skin allergies, thanks to their anti-inflammatory properties. They can also help alleviate joint pain and stiffness, offering relief for older dogs or those suffering from arthritis.

But nettle's benefits extend far beyond these. Studies have shown it can be a natural aid for respiratory problems, helping to clear congestion and ease breathing. Imagine your feline friend finally finding relief from those pesky seasonal sniffles!

- **Alfalfa:** This leafy green wonder is a natural source of protein, fiber, and essential vitamins. Alfalfa can be particularly helpful for growing puppies and kittens, providing the building blocks they need for healthy development.

Beyond its foundational benefits, alfalfa also boasts potential as a natural detoxifier. It can gently cleanse your pet's system of built-up toxins, promoting overall well-being and energy levels. Think of it as a gentle spring cleaning for your pet's internal landscape.

These are just a few examples of the incredible potential held within the world of herbal support. As you explore further, you'll discover a vast array of plants, each with its own unique set of benefits for our furry (or feathered) friends.

## Safe Supplementation: Tailoring Herbs to Your Pet

While the potential of herbal support is undeniable, it's crucial to remember that responsible pet ownership requires a measured approach. Just like medications, not all herbs are suitable for all pets. Here's what you need to consider before incorporating herbal supplements into your pet's routine:

- **Species:** A cat's needs differ greatly from a dog's. Certain herbs that are safe and beneficial for one species may be harmful to the other. Always research the specific needs of your pet's species before introducing any new herbal supplement. For instance, garlic, a common culinary herb, is considered toxic for cats but can offer some heart-healthy benefits for dogs in small, controlled amounts.

- **Size:** Just like humans, smaller pets require smaller doses of herbal supplements. A dose appropriate for a Great Dane would be far too much for a Chihuahua! Always consult the recommended dosage on the product label, and when in doubt, err on the side of caution and consult your veterinarian for guidance specific to your pet's size and breed.

- **Age:** Puppies and kittens have different needs than adult pets, and senior animals may have additional considerations. Some herbs might be too stimulating for young pets, while others could offer targeted support for aging joints in senior dogs. It's important to choose age-appropriate herbal supplements to ensure your pet receives the right kind of support at each stage of life.

- **Underlying Medical Conditions:** If your pet has any pre-existing health conditions, it's vital to discuss herbal supplementation with your veterinarian first. Certain herbs can interact with medications your pet might be taking, or could potentially exacerbate existing health issues. Your veterinarian can help you navigate these complexities and ensure herbal supplements complement, rather than hinder, your pet's current treatment plan.

**Remember:** When it comes to herbal supplements, knowledge is power. Don't hesitate to consult your veterinarian for personalized recommendations based on your pet's unique needs and medical history. They can be your trusted guide on this journey of exploring the potential of herbal support for your furry friend.

Now that we've established the importance of safe and responsible supplementation, let's get down to the fun part – **incorporating these herbal wonders into your pet's diet!**

## Brewing Up Goodness: Recipes for Delicious and Nutritious Herbal Treats

Imagine the look on your pet's face as they discover a world of delightful flavors and hidden health benefits. Here are some pawsome (or wing-tastic!) recipes featuring the herbal powerhouses we discussed earlier:

### 1. Soothing Seaweed Broth for Dogs:

This broth is a fantastic way to boost your dog's overall health and hydration. It's particularly beneficial for dogs with digestive issues or those recovering from surgery.

**Ingredients:**

- 1 tablespoon dried wakame seaweed
- 1 tablespoon dried kelp flakes
- 4 cups low-sodium chicken broth (bone broth is even better!)
- 1 bay leaf

## Instructions:

1. In a saucepan, combine the dried seaweed and bay leaf with the chicken broth.
2. Bring to a boil, then reduce heat and simmer for 15 minutes.
3. Strain the broth and let it cool completely before offering it to your dog.

## Serving Suggestion:

- For a complete meal, add a scoop of your dog's regular kibble to the cooled broth.
- You can also freeze the broth in ice cube trays and offer your dog a few cubes as a refreshing treat on a hot day.

**2. Calming Nettle Tea for Cats:**

This soothing tea can be a lifesaver for stressed or anxious cats. Nettle's anti-inflammatory properties can also provide relief for cats with itchy skin.

**Ingredients:**

- 1 teaspoon dried nettle leaves
- 1 cup boiling water

**Instructions:**

1. Steep the dried nettle leaves in the boiling water for 10 minutes.

2. Strain the tea and let it cool completely before offering it to your cat in a shallow dish.

**Serving Suggestion:**

- To encourage your cat to try the tea, place a few drops on their food bowl or a favorite toy.

- **The Power of Play:** Cats are naturally curious creatures, and sometimes a little playfulness can go a long way. Soak a small, cat-safe toy (like a crinkle ball or a feather wand) in the cooled nettle tea. The enticing scent might just pique your feline friend's interest, leading them to discover the soothing properties of the tea.

## 3. Nutritious Alfalfa Sprout Topper for All Pets:

This recipe offers a delightful and nutritious way to add a boost of vitamins, minerals, and protein to your pet's diet. Alfalfa sprouts are a fantastic source of essential nutrients for both dogs and cats.

**Ingredients:**

- 1/2 cup alfalfa seeds (organic is preferred)
- 1 jar with a sprouting lid or cheesecloth

**Instructions:**

1.  Rinse the alfalfa seeds thoroughly in a colander.

2.  Place the rinsed seeds in your sprouting jar or a clean jar covered with cheesecloth.

3.  Secure the lid or cheesecloth and rinse the seeds twice daily with fresh water.

4.  Drain well after each rinse to prevent the seeds from sitting in water.

5.  Within 3-5 days, you'll see tiny white sprouts emerge. These are your alfalfa sprouts, ready to be enjoyed!

**Serving Suggestion:**

- Sprinkle a generous handful of fresh alfalfa sprouts over your pet's regular food at mealtime.

- You can also chop the sprouts finely and mix them into homemade wet food recipes.
- Be mindful of portion size! A small handful is sufficient for most pets, with larger breeds potentially enjoying a bit more.

## Beyond the Recipes: Exploring a World of Herbal Possibilities

These recipes are just a starting point to ignite your creativity. As you delve deeper into the world of herbal support for pets, you'll discover a vast array of options to explore. Here are some additional ideas to get you thinking:

- **For Skin and Coat Health:** Consider adding herbs like dandelion root or chamomile to your pet's food. These herbs possess anti-inflammatory properties that can soothe itchy skin and promote a healthy coat.

- **For Digestive Support:** If your pet experiences occasional digestive troubles, herbs like slippery elm bark or ginger can be incorporated into their diet. These herbs have soothing properties that can ease discomfort and promote healthy digestion.

- **For Joint Health:** As pets age, joint pain can become a concern. Herbs like glucosamine and chondroitin can offer natural support for healthy joints. However, it's important to discuss these options with your veterinarian to determine the right dosage and ensure these supplements don't interact with any medications your pet might be taking.

**Remember:** When exploring new herbs, introduce them gradually to your pet's diet. Start with a very small amount and monitor for any adverse reactions. If you notice any changes in your pet's behavior, appetite, or stool, discontinue the herb and consult your veterinarian.

## A Final Note: Working with Your Veterinarian

While this chapter has explored the potential benefits of herbal support for pets, it's crucial to remember that these supplements are not a magic bullet. They should be viewed as complementary tools to enhance your pet's overall well-being, not as replacements for veterinary care.

Your veterinarian is your trusted partner in your pet's health. Before introducing any new herbal supplements into your pet's routine, discuss your intentions with your vet. They can offer valuable guidance based on your pet's unique needs and medical history.

Working together, you can create a holistic approach to pet care that incorporates the best of both traditional veterinary medicine and the potential benefits of herbal support. With knowledge, care, and a dash of creativity, you can unlock a world of natural well-being for your furry (or feathered) friend.

Remember, a happy and healthy pet is a pet who thrives on a combination of love, proper nutrition, and responsible pet ownership. By incorporating the fascinating world of herbal support into your pet's life, you can embark on a journey of holistic wellness, ensuring your cherished companion enjoys a long and fulfilling life by your side.

# Chapter 8

## Unleashing the Power of Herbs for Sparkling Smiles - A Holistic Approach to Pet Dental Health

Just like us humans, our furry (or feathered) companions require proper dental care to maintain overall health and well-being. Imagine your playful pup or curious cat with a sparkling smile and fresh breath – that's the power of good oral hygiene! This chapter delves into the fascinating world of herbal support for pet dental health.

We'll explore the incredible potential of natural ingredients like neem, clove, and cinnamon, unveiling their power to combat plaque and bacteria buildup, promote healthy gums, and contribute to a fresh, minty breath. But maintaining a pearly-white grin goes beyond just these botanical wonders.

We'll also delve into creating DIY herbal toothpastes, rinses, and chews, empowering you to pamper your pet's smile from the comfort of your own home. Think of it as a spa day for your pet's pearly whites! However, dental care isn't just about aesthetics; it's about preventing serious health concerns.

The chapter concludes by equipping you to recognize the signs of periodontal disease, a potentially debilitating condition affecting many pets. We'll explore how a holistic approach, combining the power of herbs with proper veterinary care, can address this issue and ensure your pet enjoys a lifetime of good oral health.

So, grab your metaphorical toothbrush and toothpaste, pet parents! We're about to embark on a journey of discovering how the magic of nature can contribute to a sparkling smile and a healthy mouth for your beloved companion.

## Nature's Arsenal for Sparkling Smiles: Unveiling the Power of Herbs

Maintaining good oral hygiene in our pets goes beyond simply buying fancy dental chews from the pet store. Nature provides a treasure trove of potent herbs that can be incorporated into your pet's dental care routine. Here are three powerhouses worth exploring:

- **Neem:** This versatile herb, revered in Ayurvedic medicine, boasts powerful antibacterial and antifungal properties. These properties make neem a fantastic natural ingredient for fighting plaque and gingivitis, promoting healthy gums and reducing inflammation.

Imagine incorporating neem into your pet's dental care routine! Neem oil can be diluted and used as a gentle mouthwash, or incorporated into homemade dental chews.

**Important Note:** While neem is safe for most pets in small quantities, ingestion of large amounts can be harmful. Always consult your veterinarian before incorporating neem into your pet's dental care routine, and ensure any products containing neem are specifically formulated for pets.

- **Clove:** This aromatic spice isn't just for holiday baking! Clove oil possesses natural numbing properties that can alleviate minor gum discomfort in pets. Additionally, clove boasts potent antibacterial properties, contributing to a healthy oral microbiome and combating bad breath.

While clove oil can be a fantastic addition to DIY dental care products, extreme caution is necessary. Clove oil, in concentrated forms, can be toxic to pets. Always dilute clove oil significantly before using it in any homemade dental care products, and consult your veterinarian for specific recommendations on safe dilution ratios for your pet.

- **Cinnamon:** Beyond its delightful flavor, cinnamon offers some fascinating benefits for pet dental health. Studies have shown that cinnamon possesses antibacterial properties that can help combat plaque buildup and reduce bad breath. The gentle warmth of cinnamon can also provide a soothing sensation on irritated gums.

Grinding a small amount of organic cinnamon can be a fantastic addition to your pet's food or homemade dental chews. However, cinnamon can irritate the skin and mucous membranes in some pets, so a patch test is crucial before incorporating it into their routine. Simply apply a small amount of diluted cinnamon paste to your pet's inner leg and monitor for any signs of irritation.

These are just a few examples of the incredible potential held within the world of herbal support for pet dental health. As you delve deeper, you'll discover a vast array of other herbs, each with its own unique properties that can contribute to a sparkling smile and healthy mouth for your furry friend.

## DIY Delights: Creating Herbal Toothpastes, Rinks, and Chews at Home

Now that we've explored the wonders of herbal allies for pet dental care, let's get crafty! This section empowers you to create your own DIY dental care products using these natural ingredients.

**Important Note:** Before embarking on any DIY project, consult your veterinarian to ensure the chosen herbs are safe for your specific pet. Additionally, always supervise your pet when they're using any homemade dental care products.

**Herbal Toothpaste for Sparkling Smiles:**

**Ingredients:**

- 1/2 cup organic coconut oil, softened
- 2 tablespoons baking soda (ensure it's aluminum-free)

- 2 tablespoons finely ground neem leaf powder (consult your veterinarian before using neem for your pet)
- 10 drops pet-safe peppermint essential oil (look for brands specifically formulated for pets)

**Instructions:**

1. In a clean bowl, combine the softened coconut oil and baking soda. Using a whisk or electric mixer, beat the ingredients together until light and fluffy.
2. Sift in the neem leaf powder and gently fold it into the mixture. Neem has a slightly bitter taste, so the coconut oil helps to mask it for your pet.

3. Finally, add the peppermint essential oil. Remember, a little goes a long way with essential oils! Start with just 5 drops and gradually add more if your pet tolerates the scent well.

4. Transfer the toothpaste to a small, airtight container. A repurposed travel-sized container or a small jar with a tight-fitting lid works perfectly.

5. Store the toothpaste in the refrigerator. Coconut oil solidifies at cooler temperatures, creating a consistency similar to commercial pet toothpastes.

**Top Tip:** Before introducing your pet to this new toothpaste, allow them to get familiar with the taste and scent. Simply dab a small amount on your finger and let them lick it off. Once they seem comfortable with the flavor, you can demonstrate using a pet toothbrush or a finger brush specifically designed for pets.

**Herbal Mouthwash for Fresher Breath:**

**Ingredients:**

- 1 cup boiling water
- 1 tablespoon dried peppermint leaves
- 1/4 teaspoon dried chamomile flowers (optional)

**Instructions:**

1. Steep the dried peppermint leaves and chamomile flowers (if using) in the boiling water for 10-15 minutes. Cover the container while steeping to retain

the volatile essential oils from the herbs.

2. Once steeped, strain the liquid into a clean, sealable container. Allow the rinse to cool completely before using it on your pet.

3. To use the mouthwash, dilute it with an equal amount of water. You can use an oral syringe or a small cup to gently administer the diluted rinse to your pet's mouth. Avoid directly squirting the rinse down their throat, as this can cause them to choke.

**Herbal Chews for Satisfying Chomps:**

**Ingredients:**

- 1 cup rolled oats
- 1/2 cup mashed sweet potato

- 1/4 cup unsweetened applesauce
- 1 tablespoon ground flaxseed
- 1 teaspoon ground cinnamon (patch test your pet before using)
- 1/2 teaspoon dried parsley flakes

**Instructions:**

1. Preheat your oven to 350°F (175°C). Line a baking sheet with parchment paper.
2. In a large bowl, combine the rolled oats, mashed sweet potato, and applesauce. Mix well to form a sticky dough.
3. Incorporate the ground flaxseed, cinnamon (if using after a patch test), and parsley flakes. Mix until evenly distributed.

4. Using your hands, form the dough into small bite-sized chews. Place them on the prepared baking sheet, leaving some space between each chew for even baking.

5. Bake the chews for 15-20 minutes, or until they become firm to the touch. Allow them to cool completely before offering them to your pet.

6. Store leftover chews in an airtight container in the refrigerator for up to a week.

**Remember:** These are just a few DIY recipe ideas to get you started. As you explore the world of herbal pet care, you'll discover a vast array of other ingredients you can incorporate into your homemade dental care products. Always prioritize safety by consulting your veterinarian before introducing any new herbs, and ensure you use pet-safe essential oils when incorporating them into your recipes.

## Beyond DIY Delights: Professional Products and Veterinary Care

While DIY dental care products can be a fantastic way to incorporate the power of herbs into your pet's routine, they shouldn't replace professional dental cleanings performed by your veterinarian. Regular dental checkups are crucial for identifying and addressing any underlying dental concerns before they progress into more serious issues.

During a dental cleaning, your veterinarian will thoroughly examine your pet's mouth, scaling away tartar buildup and cleaning below the gum line where brushing alone can't reach. They can also address any potential dental problems like loose teeth, gingivitis, or periodontal disease.

Think of professional dental cleanings as the deep cleaning your pet's smile deserves! Combined with a consistent at-home dental care routine that incorporates the power of herbs, you can ensure your pet enjoys a lifetime of ...sparkling teeth, fresh breath, and optimal oral health. This translates to a happier and healthier pet, free from the discomfort and potential health complications associated with neglected dental hygiene.

## Understanding Periodontal Disease: Recognizing the Signs and Taking a Holistic Approach

Just like humans, pets can develop periodontal disease, a serious infection of the gums and tissues surrounding the teeth. Left untreated, periodontal disease can lead to significant pain, tooth loss, and even systemic health problems like heart disease.

**Early Detection is Key:** The good news is that periodontal disease is preventable and treatable, especially when detected in its early stages. Here are some signs to watch out for in your pet:

- **Bad breath:** This is a classic sign of dental problems, including periodontal disease. While occasional bad breath is normal, persistent foul odor emanating from your pet's mouth warrants a visit to the veterinarian.

- **Red, swollen, or bleeding gums:** Healthy gums should be pink and firm. Redness, swelling, or bleeding gums indicate inflammation and potential infection.
- **Loose teeth:** Periodontal disease can weaken the supporting structures around the teeth, leading to loose or wobbly teeth.
- **Difficulty chewing:** Pain associated with inflamed gums or loose teeth can make chewing uncomfortable for your pet. They might shy away from hard kibble or seem hesitant to chew on their favorite toys.

- **Drooling:** Excessive drooling can be a sign of dental pain or discomfort.

## A Holistic Approach to Periodontal Disease:

If you notice any of these signs in your pet, schedule an appointment with your veterinarian right away. Early diagnosis and treatment are crucial for preventing further progression of the disease.

In addition to veterinary treatment, a holistic approach that incorporates the power of herbs can play a supportive role in managing periodontal disease. Here's how:

- **Herbal Mouthwashes:** As discussed earlier, herbal mouthwashes made with peppermint or chamomile can help freshen breath and soothe inflamed gums.

- **Antibacterial Herbs:** Certain herbs like neem and clove possess natural antibacterial properties. Consulting your veterinarian, you can explore incorporating these herbs (in safe quantities) into your pet's diet or dental care routine to combat the bacteria that contribute to periodontal disease.

- **Immune-Supporting Herbs:** A healthy immune system is essential for fighting off infection. Astragalus and Echinacea are two herbs known for their immune-modulating properties. However, it's crucial to discuss these herbs with your veterinarian before introducing them to your pet, as they can interact with certain medications.

**Remember:** Herbal remedies should be viewed as complementary to veterinary treatment for periodontal disease, not a replacement. Early diagnosis, professional dental cleanings, and appropriate antibiotics are essential for effectively managing this condition.

## Conclusion: A Winning Smile for Life

By incorporating the power of herbs into your pet's dental care routine, combined with regular veterinary checkups and professional cleanings, you can empower your furry (or feathered) friend to maintain a sparkling smile and optimal oral health for a lifetime. Think of it as an investment in their overall well-being, ensuring they enjoy a pain-free mouth, fresh breath, and the ability to savor their favorite treats for years to come.

So, the next time you cuddle with your beloved pet, take a moment to appreciate their pearly whites (or perhaps their sharp little canines!). With a little proactive care and the magic of natural herbs, you can ensure their smile stays healthy and happy for a lifetime of love, laughter, and playful chomps.

# Chapter 9

## The Wonder Years: Nurturing the Health and Happiness of Your Puppy or Kitten

Welcoming a playful puppy or a curious kitten into your life is an experience brimming with joy, laughter, and unconditional love. However, along with the overflowing cuteness comes the responsibility of ensuring their health and well-being during this crucial developmental stage. This chapter serves as your guide to navigating the "wonder years" of your furry (or feathered) friend, equipping you with the knowledge and tools to foster their optimal growth and development.

Here, we'll delve into the intricacies of proper medication and supplement dosing specifically for puppies and kittens. We'll explore the potential of certain herbs to support their development, immune function, and digestion. Additionally, we'll address common behavioral concerns like separation anxiety and house training, offering holistic approaches to manage these challenges effectively.

Remember, this chapter is not intended as a substitute for professional veterinary advice. Always consult your veterinarian before administering any medication, supplements, or introducing new herbs into your pet's routine.

Think of this chapter as a roadmap, empowering you to ask informed questions during your veterinary visits and work collaboratively with your vet to create a personalized healthcare plan tailored to your precious puppy or kitten's unique needs.

## Dosage Dilemmas: Ensuring Safe and Effective Medication Administration

Puppies and kittens are not simply miniature versions of adult dogs and cats. Their bodies are undergoing rapid development, and their metabolisms work differently than those of their fully grown counterparts. This has a significant impact on how medications and supplements are processed and eliminated from their bodies. Here's why proper dosing is crucial:

- **Safety First:** Administering an incorrect dose of medication can have serious consequences for your young pet. A dose that might be safe for an adult animal could be potentially toxic to a developing puppy or kitten.

- **Efficacy Matters:** An under-dose might not be effective in treating the intended condition, leaving your pet vulnerable to illness. Conversely, an over-dose might not provide any additional benefit and could lead to unwanted side effects.

**The Golden Rule:** Never attempt to guesstimate a dosage for your puppy or kitten. Always rely on the expertise of your veterinarian to determine the correct amount of medication based on your pet's weight, age, and overall health.

Here are some additional tips for safe and effective medication administration:

- **Read the Label Carefully:** Before administering any medication, thoroughly read the label and follow the instructions precisely. Pay close attention to the dosage amount, frequency of administration, and any potential side effects.

- **Liquid Medications:** If administering liquid medication, use the measuring device provided (such as a dropper or syringe) and ensure you're measuring the exact amount prescribed.

- **Tablets and Capsules:** For tablets and capsules, consult your veterinarian on the best way to administer them to your pet. Some medications might need to be crushed and mixed with food, while others can be given whole.

- **Observe Your Pet:** After administering any medication, monitor your pet for any signs of adverse reactions like vomiting, diarrhea, or lethargy. If you notice any concerning symptoms, contact your veterinarian immediately.

By following these guidelines and working closely with your veterinarian, you can ensure your puppy or kitten receives the proper medication dosage for optimal treatment and remains safe throughout the process.

## Herbal Allies for Thriving Pups and Kittens: Supporting Development, Immunity, and Digestion

Nature offers a treasure trove of potential allies to support the well-being of your growing puppy or kitten. Here's a glimpse into the world of herbs that can be particularly beneficial during this crucial developmental stage:

- **Nurturing Development:** Milk thistle, a revered herb with antioxidant and liver-protective properties, can be particularly beneficial for puppies and kittens. Their rapidly developing bodies require a significant amount of nutrients for healthy growth. Milk thistle can potentially support their liver function, which plays a vital role in processing these essential nutrients. Important Note: Always consult your veterinarian before introducing milk thistle to your puppy or kitten, as it can interact with certain medications.

- **Boosting Immunity:** Echinacea, a popular herb known for its potential immune-modulating properties, might offer gentle support for your puppy or kitten's developing immune system. Consult your veterinarian to determine if introducing Echinacea (specifically formulated for pets) into your pet's routine is appropriate, especially during times of stress or potential exposure to illness.

- **Aiding Digestion:** Probiotics are live microorganisms that can be incredibly beneficial for gut health, especially in young puppies and kittens. Their digestive systems are still maturing, and probiotics can help establish a healthy balance of gut flora, potentially promoting smoother digestion and reducing the likelihood of gastrointestinal upset. Consider discussing the possibility of incorporating a pet-specific probiotic supplement into your puppy or kitten's routine with your veterinarian.

**Remember:** Herbs are not a replacement for proper nutrition and veterinary care. Always consult your veterinarian before introducing any new herbs into your pet's routine, and ensure they are specifically formulated for use in puppies or kittens.

While research on the efficacy of herbs in young pets is ongoing, these natural allies hold promise for offering gentle support during their crucial developmental stages. However, it's crucial to approach them with a measured perspective. Open communication with your veterinarian is key to determining the most appropriate approach for your specific pet's needs.

## Beyond Cute Chewing: Holistic Approaches to Behavioral Challenges

Welcoming a new puppy or kitten into your life brings immense joy, however, it can also come with some behavioral challenges. Separation anxiety and house-training difficulties are two common concerns new pet parents face. Let's explore holistic approaches to address these challenges effectively:

- **Conquering Separation Anxiety:** Separation anxiety can manifest in a variety of ways, including destructive chewing, excessive barking or meowing, and pacing. Here are some holistic strategies to help your puppy or kitten feel secure and comfortable in your absence:

- **Gradual Desensitization:** Start by leaving your pet alone for short periods of time and gradually increase the duration as they become more comfortable. Pair your departures with positive reinforcement, like offering a favorite toy or treat before you leave.

- **Creating a Safe Space:** Provide your puppy or kitten with a designated safe space, like a crate or a comfortable playpen, where they feel secure and content when you're not around.

Ensure this space is filled with familiar toys and bedding.

- **Mental Stimulation:** Before leaving, engage your pet in a stimulating activity like a short play session or a food puzzle challenge. This can help tire them out and create a positive association with your departure.

- **House-Training with Heart:** House-training requires patience and consistency. Here are some holistic tips to help your puppy or kitten learn the desired potty etiquette:

  - **Establish a Routine:** Take your puppy or kitten outside frequently, especially after meals, playtime, or waking up from sleep. Consistency is key in helping them understand where and when it's appropriate to eliminate.

- ○ **Positive Reinforcement:** When your pet eliminates outdoors, praise them lavishly and offer a small treat. This positive reinforcement helps them associate going potty outside with a reward.

- ○ **Accident Management:** Accidents happen, especially during the learning process. When your pet has an accident, clean the area thoroughly with an enzymatic cleaner to remove any lingering odors that might attract them to eliminate in the same spot again. Avoid punishing your pet, as this can create anxiety and hinder the learning process.

**Remember:** Patience and understanding are crucial when addressing behavioral challenges in your young pet. Holistic approaches, combined with consistent positive reinforcement training, can help your puppy or kitten develop the desired behaviors and live a happy, well-adjusted life.

## Building a Foundation for Lifelong Wellness: The Importance of Preventative Care

The first few months of life are a critical window for establishing healthy habits that will benefit your puppy or kitten throughout their lives. Preventative care plays a pivotal role in this process. Here's why:

- **Vaccinations and Parasite Prevention:** Puppies and kittens require a series of vaccinations to protect them from potentially life-threatening diseases. Additionally, regular parasite prevention medication is crucial to safeguard them from internal and external parasites. Discuss a comprehensive vaccination and parasite prevention plan with your veterinarian to ensure your pet receives the necessary protection.

- **Early Socialization:** Socialization is the process of exposing your puppy or kitten to a variety of people, animals, and environments in a positive and controlled manner. Early socialization helps them develop confidence, reduce fearfulness, and become well-adjusted companions. Enroll your puppy or kitten in puppy socialization classes or kitten socialization sessions offered by qualified trainers or animal shelters.

- **Nutritional Support:** Proper nutrition is essential for optimal growth and development in puppies and kittens. Discuss with your veterinarian the best type of food to feed your pet based on their breed, age, and activity level. Choose high-quality pet food formulated specifically for puppies or kittens to ensure they receive all the essential nutrients they need to thrive.

By prioritizing preventative care, you're not only safeguarding your pet's health but also laying the foundation for a long and happy life together.

This chapter has hopefully equipped you with the knowledge and tools to navigate the "wonder years" of your puppy or kitten with confidence.

# Chapter 10

## **Navigating the Emotional Landscape: Understanding and Addressing Behavioral Issues in Pets**

The human-animal bond is a powerful and complex relationship. Our furry (or feathered) companions offer us unconditional love, companionship, and a sense of purpose. However, just like us, pets can experience a range of emotions, and sometimes, these emotions can manifest in ways that we find challenging. This chapter delves into the world of pet behavior, equipping you to understand the root causes of emotional and behavioral issues and explore various strategies to address them effectively.

Here, we'll explore the potential of specific herbs to gently support pets struggling with reactivity, fear, obsessive behaviors, and more. We'll delve into the power of environmental enrichment, pheromones, and positive reinforcement training in modifying unwanted behaviors. Finally, we'll emphasize the importance of fostering a strong human-animal bond through massage, play therapy, and establishing a consistent routine, creating a foundation for emotional well-being in your pet.

Remember, this chapter is not intended as a substitute for professional veterinary or animal behaviorist advice. If you're concerned about your pet's emotional or behavioral well-being, always consult with a qualified professional to develop a personalized plan tailored to your pet's specific needs. Think of us as embarking on a journey together, where you gain the knowledge and tools to navigate your pet's emotional landscape and create a harmonious relationship.

## Herbal Allies for Emotional Harmony: Supporting Calmness and Well-being

While herbs are not a magic bullet for behavioral issues, certain herbs can potentially offer gentle support for pets experiencing emotional distress. Here's a glimpse into some options to consider:

- **Promoting Calmness:** Chamomile, a revered herb known for its calming properties, might be beneficial for pets exhibiting signs of anxiety or hyperactivity. Chamomile tea (cooled and offered in a shallow dish) or chamomile supplements (specifically formulated for pets) can potentially promote relaxation and reduce stress. Important Note: Consult your veterinarian before introducing chamomile to your pet, as it can interact with certain medications.

- **Addressing Fear:** Valerian root, an herb with historical use as a natural sedative, might offer some relief for pets experiencing fear-based behaviors, such as separation anxiety or noise phobias. However, research on its effectiveness in pets is ongoing.

Discuss with your veterinarian if incorporating Valerian root supplements (formulated for pets) into your pet's routine might be a suitable approach.

- **Curbing Obsessions:** While research is limited, some pet owners have reported success in using L-theanine, an amino acid found in green tea, to manage obsessive behaviors in their pets. L-theanine is thought to promote relaxation and focus. Consult your veterinarian to determine if L-theanine supplements (formulated for pets) could be a potential option for your pet.

**Remember:** Always introduce herbs gradually and monitor your pet for any adverse reactions. Herbs should never be used as a replacement for veterinary treatment or behavior modification techniques.

**A Word of Caution:** Several herbs and essential oils can be toxic to pets. Never administer essential oils directly to your pet, and avoid using diffusers in their vicinity. Always consult your veterinarian before introducing any new herbs or supplements into your pet's routine.

## Environmental Enrichment: Creating a World of Stimulation

Our pets are complex creatures with a natural desire to explore and engage with their environment. A lack of environmental enrichment can lead to boredom, frustration, and the development of unwanted behaviors. Here are some strategies to create a stimulating environment for your pet:

- **Interactive Toys:** Provide your pet with a variety of interactive toys that challenge their minds and encourage problem-solving skills. Rotate the toys regularly to maintain their interest. Food puzzles that dispense treats as your pet works for them are a great way to combine mental stimulation with a tasty reward.

- **Species-Specific Enrichment:** Cater to your pet's natural instincts.

For cats, provide scratching posts, climbing structures, and window perches for birdwatching. For dogs, offer snuffle mats to encourage foraging behaviors, and consider puzzle feeders to slow down their eating and engage their minds.

- **Outdoor Exploration:** For dogs that enjoy it, regular walks and outdoor adventures provide essential mental and physical stimulation. Sniffing new scents, exploring different environments, and engaging in physical activity can all contribute to your dog's emotional well-being.

**Remember:** Environmental enrichment is an ongoing process. Continuously evaluate your pet's needs and preferences and introduce new enrichment activities to keep them engaged and prevent boredom.

## Harnessing the Power of Pheromones and Positive Reinforcement Training

Pheromones are natural chemical signals used by animals for communication. While pheromones might not be a cure-all for behavioral issues, they can be a valuable tool when used in conjunction with other strategies. Here's how:

- **Calming Signals:** Synthetic versions of canine appeasing pheromones (CAP) are available commercially. These pheromones mimic the natural calming signals produced by lactating mothers. Diffusing CAP in your home can potentially create a more relaxing environment for your dog, particularly helpful during stressful situations like thunderstorms or fireworks displays.

- **Confidence Boosters:** For shy or fearful dogs, synthetic dog appeasing pheromones (DAP) can be applied to a collar or bandana worn by the dog. These pheromones might help promote feelings of security and confidence, making them more receptive to training and less likely to react fearfully in new situations.

**Important Note:** Pheromones are not a quick fix. Their effectiveness can vary depending on the individual pet and the severity of the behavioral issue. Always consult with your veterinarian or a qualified animal behaviorist to determine if pheromones could be a beneficial addition to your pet's treatment plan.

## Positive Reinforcement Training:

Positive reinforcement training is a humane and effective method for modifying unwanted behaviors and teaching your pet new ones. This approach focuses on rewarding desired behaviors with treats, praise, or playtime. Here are some key principles:

- **Reward the Right Behavior:** Only reward the behavior you want to see. For example, if your dog is barking incessantly, wait for a quiet moment and then reward them calmly for being quiet.

- **Consistency is Key:** Positive reinforcement training requires consistency from you. Use clear commands, reward desired behaviors promptly, and avoid using punishment or harsh corrections.

- **Patience is a Virtue:** Learning takes time. Be patient with your pet and celebrate small successes along the way. Positive reinforcement training can be a rewarding experience for both you and your pet, strengthening your bond and creating a more harmonious relationship.

**Remember:** Positive reinforcement training is an ongoing process. Regular practice and consistency are key to achieving lasting results. If you're facing significant behavioral challenges, consider seeking guidance from a certified professional animal trainer.

## The Magic Touch: Fostering the Human-Animal Bond Through Massage and Play

The human-animal bond is a powerful force that can significantly influence your pet's emotional well-being. Here are some ways to strengthen this bond and promote emotional harmony:

- **The Power of Massage:** Pet massage can be a wonderful way to relax your pet, reduce stress, and strengthen your connection. Learn basic massage techniques from a qualified professional or veterinarian and incorporate gentle massage sessions into your pet's regular routine.

- **Play Therapy:** Play is not just about fun; it's essential for your pet's physical and mental well-being. Engage in daily play sessions with your pet, tailoring activities to their age, energy level, and preferences. Interactive games like fetch, tug-of-war, or puzzle toys can all contribute to a happy and well-adjusted pet.

- **Routine and Rituals:** Pets thrive on routine. Establishing consistent feeding times, walk schedules, and playtime sessions creates a sense of security and predictability for them. Additionally, incorporate positive rituals into your daily routine, such as a gentle head scratch before bed or a cuddle session on the couch. These rituals create positive associations and strengthen the bond between you and your pet.

By incorporating these strategies into your daily life, you can create a nurturing environment that fosters your pet's emotional well-being. Remember, a strong human-animal bond is the foundation for a happy and fulfilling life for both you and your furry (or feathered) companion.

**Remember:** Understanding your pet's emotional needs and addressing behavioral issues with a holistic approach can significantly improve their quality of life and strengthen the bond you share. If you're ever unsure about how to address a specific behavioral concern, don't hesitate to consult your veterinarian or a qualified animal behaviorist. Together, you can create a harmonious and enriching environment for your cherished pet.

# Chapter 11

## Safeguarding the Engine: Promoting Cardiovascular Health in Pets

The heart, a tireless pump propelling life-giving blood throughout the body, plays a pivotal role in your pet's overall health and well-being. Just like us, pets can develop cardiovascular concerns that can significantly impact their quality of life. This chapter delves into the world of pet cardiology, empowering you to understand the importance of maintaining a healthy heart in your furry (or feathered) companion.

Here, we'll explore the potential of certain herbs to support circulation and cardiac function. We'll delve into the power of diet and lifestyle modifications in preventing or managing heart disease in pets. Additionally, we'll equip you to recognize the warning signs of cardiovascular trouble, encouraging you to seek prompt veterinary attention for your pet if necessary.

Remember, this chapter is not intended as a substitute for professional veterinary advice. If you have any concerns about your pet's heart health, schedule an appointment with your veterinarian for a thorough evaluation. Think of us as embarking on a journey together, where you gain the knowledge and tools to become a proactive advocate for your pet's cardiovascular well-being.

## Herbal Allies for a Strong Heart: Supporting Circulation and Function

While herbs are not a replacement for veterinary treatment for established heart disease, certain herbs have shown promise in supporting healthy circulation and cardiac function. Here's a glimpse into some options to consider:

- **Hawthorn Berry**: This revered herb has a long history of use in traditional European medicine for heart health. Hawthorn berries may help improve circulation by strengthening blood vessel walls and increasing blood flow. Important Note: Consult your veterinarian before introducing hawthorn berry to your pet, as it can interact with certain medications.

- **Ginkgo Biloba:** This ancient herb is known for its potential benefits on circulation. Ginkgo biloba might help improve blood flow, particularly to the brain, potentially enhancing cognitive function in senior pets. Important Note: Research on the effectiveness of Ginkgo biloba in pets is ongoing. Discuss with your veterinarian if it could be a suitable option for your pet.

**Remember:** Always introduce herbs gradually and monitor your pet for any adverse reactions. Herbs should never be used as a substitute for veterinary treatment or a well-balanced diet. It's crucial to consult your veterinarian before incorporating any new herbs into your pet's routine to ensure their safety and suitability.

**A Word of Caution:** Several herbs and essential oils can be toxic to pets. Never administer essential oils directly to your pet, and avoid using diffusers in their vicinity.

## Diet and Lifestyle: The Pillars of a Healthy Heart

Just like in humans, diet and lifestyle play a crucial role in promoting cardiovascular health in pets. Here's how you can make a difference:

- **Nutritional Support:** A balanced and species-appropriate diet is essential for optimal heart health. Discuss with your veterinarian the best food to feed your pet based on their age, breed, activity level, and any existing health conditions. Look for pet foods formulated with ingredients that support heart health, such as omega-3 fatty acids, L-carnitine, and antioxidants.

- **Weight Management:** Obesity is a significant risk factor for heart disease in pets. Maintaining your pet at a healthy weight can significantly reduce the strain on their heart. Work with your veterinarian to develop a weight management plan if your pet is overweight or obese. This might involve slight adjustments to portion sizes, increased exercise opportunities, or switching to a weight-management diet formulated for pets.

- **Exercise for Every Heart:** Regular exercise is crucial for maintaining a healthy heart in pets. The type and intensity of exercise will vary depending on your pet's age, breed, and overall health. Consult your veterinarian for guidance on creating a safe and effective exercise routine for your pet.

**Remember:** Consistency is key! Aim for daily walks, playtime sessions, or other forms of exercise tailored to your pet's preferences and abilities.

# Recognizing the Signs of Heart Trouble: Early Detection Saves Lives

Just like us, pets can't tell us verbally when they're not feeling well. Being observant and recognizing the subtle signs of potential heart trouble in your pet can make a world of difference. Here's what to watch out for:

- **Decreased Exercise Tolerance:** If your pet tires easily during walks or playtime, it could be a sign of reduced heart function. Pay attention to their energy levels and any reluctance to engage in activities they typically enjoy.

- **Coughing or Difficulty Breathing:** A persistent cough, especially at night or when resting, can be a symptom of heart disease in pets. Difficulty breathing, rapid panting (even at rest), or excessive panting during mild activity are also cause for concern.

- **Lethargy and Weakness:** If your pet seems unusually lethargic, weak, or disinterested in activities they normally enjoy, it could be a sign of an underlying health condition, including heart disease.

- **Pale Gums:** Healthy gums should be a pink color. Pale or white gums can indicate poor circulation, which could be a sign of heart trouble.

- **Abdominal Distention:** Fluid accumulation in the abdomen (ascites) can occur in pets with advanced heart disease. If your pet's abdomen appears swollen or distended, prompt veterinary attention is crucial.

**Remember:** Early detection and treatment are essential for managing heart disease effectively and improving your pet's quality of life. If you notice any of these signs in your pet, don't hesitate to schedule an appointment with your veterinarian for a thorough evaluation.

## Seeking Veterinary Care: Prompt Action for a Healthy Future

If you suspect your pet might be experiencing heart trouble, seeking prompt veterinary care is crucial. Here's what to expect:

- **Diagnostic Tests:** Your veterinarian might recommend various tests to diagnose heart disease, such as X-rays, electrocardiograms (ECGs), and echocardiograms. These tests can help assess your pet's heart function and identify any structural abnormalities.

- **Treatment Options:** The treatment plan for your pet's heart disease will depend on the severity of the condition and the underlying cause.

Treatment options might include medication, dietary modifications, and lifestyle changes. In some cases, minimally invasive procedures or surgery might be necessary.

**Remember:** Your veterinarian is your partner in safeguarding your pet's heart health. Work collaboratively with them to develop a treatment plan tailored to your pet's specific needs and provide them with the love, support, and care they need to thrive.

## Living with Heart Disease: Enhancing Your Pet's Quality of Life

A diagnosis of heart disease doesn't have to mean the end of a happy and fulfilling life for your pet. With proper management and care, pets with heart disease can live long and relatively healthy lives. Here's how you can help:

- **Medication Adherence:** If your pet is prescribed medication for heart disease, it's crucial to administer it consistently and according to your veterinarian's instructions. Missing doses can compromise the effectiveness of the medication.

- **Maintaining a Healthy Weight:** Weight management remains crucial for pets with heart disease. Continue working with your veterinarian to ensure your pet stays at a healthy weight to minimize the strain on their heart.

- **Exercise with Caution:** While exercise is essential for overall health, it's important to adjust the intensity and duration of your pet's exercise routine based on their veterinarian's recommendations. Avoid strenuous activity that could put undue stress on their heart.

- **Regular Checkups:** Schedule regular follow-up appointments with your veterinarian to monitor your pet's heart health and adjust treatment as needed. Early detection of any changes can help prevent complications and improve your pet's quality of life.

**Remember:** With love, care, and a proactive approach, you can help your pet with heart disease live a long and happy life. Don't hesitate to reach out to your veterinarian for guidance and support along the way.

By understanding the importance of cardiovascular health in pets, implementing preventative measures, and recognizing the warning signs of potential trouble, you can become a champion for your pet's heart health. Remember, early detection and prompt veterinary intervention are key to ensuring your furry (or feathered) companion enjoys a long and healthy life by your side.

# Chapter 12

## Navigating the Journey: Supporting Your Pet with Cancer

A cancer diagnosis for a beloved pet can be a deeply emotional experience. Many pet parents feel overwhelmed and unsure of how to best support their furry (or feathered) companion throughout their treatment journey. This chapter serves as a beacon of hope, outlining ways to integrate complementary therapies alongside conventional veterinary treatment to bolster your pet's well-being and potentially improve their quality of life.

Here, we'll delve into the potential of herbs to mitigate common side effects associated with cancer treatment, like pain, nausea, and anxiety. We'll explore the fascinating world of medicinal mushrooms and antioxidants, unveiling their potential role in supporting the body's natural defenses.

But this journey extends beyond just supplements. We'll also explore the power of lifestyle and nutritive therapies, emphasizing the importance of nutrition, exercise, and stress management in supporting your pet's overall vitality and comfort.

Remember, this chapter is not intended as a substitute for professional veterinary advice. Always consult with your veterinarian before introducing any new supplements or making changes to your pet's treatment plan. Think of this chapter as a roadmap, empowering you to discuss these complementary therapies with your veterinarian and create a holistic approach tailored to your pet's unique needs.

## Herbal Allies: Mitigating the Side Effects of Treatment

Cancer treatment, while life-saving, can often come with a range of side effects. Nausea, vomiting, pain, and anxiety are some of the most common concerns pet parents face. Here's how certain herbs can potentially offer gentle support:

- **Calming the Anxious Mind:** A cancer diagnosis can be stressful for both pets and their owners. Herbs like chamomile and lavender possess calming properties that can help ease anxiety and promote relaxation. Consider adding a chamomile tea (made specifically for pets, not humans!) to your pet's water bowl, or diffusing diluted lavender essential oil in a pet-safe diffuser to create a calming environment.

**Important Note:** Essential oils can be very potent, and some can be toxic to pets. Always choose pet-safe essential oils specifically formulated for aromatherapy use in animals, and dilute them properly before diffusing them in a pet-safe diffuser.

- **Taming the Tummy Troubles:** Nausea and vomiting are common side effects of certain cancer treatments. Ginger root is a well-known natural remedy for nausea, and some studies suggest it can be effective in mitigating nausea in pets as well. Consult your veterinarian about incorporating ginger into your pet's diet, either in small, grated pieces or as a ginger tea specifically formulated for pets.

- **Soothing the Ache:** Managing pain is crucial for your pet's comfort throughout their treatment journey. Certain herbs, like turmeric and curcumin, possess anti-inflammatory properties that may help alleviate pain. Discuss with your veterinarian the possibility of incorporating turmeric or curcumin supplements into your pet's routine, ensuring they are formulated specifically for pets and appropriate for their individual needs.

**Remember:** Herbs are not meant to replace pain medications prescribed by your veterinarian. They can, however, offer gentle support and potentially reduce the reliance on pain medication.

It's important to note that the research on the efficacy of herbs in pets with cancer is still ongoing. While some studies show promising results, more research is needed to definitively determine the best herbal protocols for specific types of cancer and their side effects.

The key takeaway? Open communication with your veterinarian is essential. Discuss the potential benefits and drawbacks of incorporating specific herbs into your pet's treatment plan, ensuring they won't interact with any medications your pet might already be taking.

## The Power of Medicinal Mushrooms and Antioxidants: Boosting the Body's Defenses

Nature offers a treasure trove of potent allies beyond traditional herbs. Medicinal mushrooms and antioxidants have emerged as exciting areas of research in the fight against cancer. Let's explore their potential:

- **Medicinal Mushrooms:** These fascinating fungi have been used in traditional medicine for centuries, and recent research suggests they may play a role in supporting the body's immune system during cancer treatment. Mushrooms like Reishi, Shiitake, and Maitake possess immunomodulatory properties, meaning they can help regulate the immune system and potentially enhance its ability to fight cancer cells.

**Important Note:** Medicinal mushrooms can interact with certain medications. Always consult with your veterinarian before introducing any medicinal mushrooms into your pet's diet.

- Antioxidant Arsenal: Cancer cells thrive in an environment with high levels of free radicals. Antioxidants act as nature's "scavengers," neutralizing these free radicals and protecting healthy cells from damage. Fruits rich in antioxidants like blueberries, cranberries, and pomegranates can be incorporated into your pet's diet (in moderation

(in moderation, of course) to contribute to their overall antioxidant intake. Similarly, vegetables like broccoli, carrots, and leafy greens are packed with antioxidant power. Discuss with your veterinarian the possibility of adding these antioxidant-rich foods to your pet's diet in a way that complements their existing food plan.

A Note on Caution: While medicinal mushrooms and antioxidants hold promise, it's crucial to approach them with a measured perspective. More research is needed to definitively determine their efficacy in treating cancer in pets. They should never be viewed as a replacement for conventional veterinary treatment. Think of them as potential allies in your pet's fight, but always work closely with your veterinarian to integrate them safely and effectively.

Beyond Supplements: Lifestyle and Nutritive Therapies for Optimal Wellbeing

While herbs, mushrooms, and antioxidants can offer valuable support, a holistic approach to caring for your pet with cancer extends far beyond supplements. Lifestyle and nutritive therapies play a crucial role in promoting vitality, managing symptoms, and enhancing your pet's overall quality of life. Let's delve deeper:

- The Power of Nutrition: Nutrition is the foundation of health, and this is especially true for pets battling cancer. A balanced diet rich in essential nutrients can help support your pet's immune system, promote healing, and manage their energy levels. Discuss with your veterinarian the possibility of switching your pet to a high-quality diet specifically formulated for pets with cancer. These diets often prioritize easily digestible ingredients, increased protein content to support tissue repair, and optimal levels of omega-3 fatty acids, which possess anti-inflammatory properties.

Remember: Not all commercially available "cancer" diets are created equal. Work with your veterinarian to choose a diet that meets your pet's specific needs and preferences.

- Maintaining a Healthy Weight: Obesity can negatively impact a pet's overall health and potentially hinder cancer treatment. If your pet is overweight, work with your veterinarian to develop a safe and gradual weight loss plan. This might involve slight adjustments to portion sizes, increased exercise opportunities, or switching to a weight-management diet formulated for pets.

- The Importance of Exercise: While your pet might experience reduced energy levels during treatment, gentle exercise is crucial for maintaining muscle mass, improving mood, and promoting overall well-being. Tailor your pet's exercise routine to their current capabilities. Short walks, playtime with a favorite toy, or even gentle swimming sessions can all contribute to their physical and mental well-being.

- Stress Management for Serenity: Cancer and its treatment can be stressful for both pets and their owners. Creating a calm and stress-free environment for your pet is essential. Minimize loud noises or unfamiliar visitors, provide ample opportunities for quiet rest, and dedicate time for gentle petting and affection. Techniques like pheromone therapy or calming music can also create a more relaxed atmosphere for your pet.

Remember: Every pet is an individual, and their needs will vary throughout their cancer journey. Open communication with your veterinarian is key to tailoring a holistic approach that prioritizes your pet's comfort and well-being. Don't hesitate to ask questions, voice your concerns, and work collaboratively with your veterinary team to create the best possible support system for your furry friend.

This chapter has hopefully shed light on the potential of complementary therapies alongside conventional veterinary treatment for pets battling cancer. While these therapies are not a cure, they can offer valuable support in managing side effects, boosting the body's defenses, and enhancing your pet's quality of life.

Remember, navigating a cancer diagnosis for a beloved pet can be emotionally challenging. Seek support from friends, family, and online communities dedicated to pet cancer care. There are also pet hospices and palliative care services available that can provide guidance and emotional support throughout this difficult journey.

The human-animal bond is truly special, and during times of illness, this connection becomes even more profound. By integrating complementary therapies with conventional veterinary treatment, and prioritizing your pet's comfort and well-being, you can embark on this journey with love, hope, and the unwavering commitment to provide your furry (or feathered) companion with the best possible care.

## Chapter 10: Silver Spoons & Golden Years: Enriching the Lives of Our Senior Pets

Our beloved furry (or feathered) companions grace our lives with unconditional love, playful antics, and a comforting presence. As they age, the roles might gently reverse. We, their devoted pet parents, become responsible for ensuring their golden years are filled with comfort, vitality, and a sense of well-being. This chapter delves into the fascinating world of senior pet care, empowering you to navigate this special time with knowledge and compassion.

Here, we'll explore the potential of specific herbs to gently support organ function, cognitive health, and mobility in our senior pets. We'll unveil some creative recipes and natural remedies tailored to their specific needs, making healthy living a delicious and engaging experience.

But senior pet care extends beyond herbal allies and tasty treats. We'll emphasize the importance of preventative care through nutritional support and routine wellness exams. By proactively addressing potential health concerns, we can ensure our senior companions enjoy a longer and healthier twilight of their lives.

So, grab your metaphorical walking stick (for those of you with senior canine companions, of course!), and let's embark on a journey of enriching the lives of our cherished senior pets!

## Herbal Allies for a Vibrant Senior Life: Supporting Organs, Mind, and Mobility

As our pets age, their bodies undergo a series of changes. Their once boundless energy levels might decrease, and certain organ functions might become less efficient. Here's how specific herbs can potentially offer gentle support:

- **Supporting Organ Function:** Milk thistle, a revered herb in traditional medicine, possesses potent antioxidant and liver-protective properties. Consider incorporating milk thistle supplements (specifically formulated for pets) into your senior pet's routine to support healthy liver function. **Important Note:** Consult your veterinarian before introducing milk thistle, as it can interact with certain medications.

- **Sharpening the Senior Mind:** Age-related cognitive decline can be a concern for many pet parents. Ginkgo biloba, an herb with a long history of use in traditional Chinese medicine, has been shown to improve cognitive function in some studies. While research on its effectiveness in pets is ongoing, discuss with your veterinarian the possibility of incorporating Ginkgo biloba supplements (formulated for pets) into your senior pet's routine, particularly if you notice any signs of cognitive decline.

- **Maintaining Mobility:** Joint pain and stiffness are common concerns in senior pets. Curcumin, the active ingredient in turmeric, possesses anti-inflammatory properties that can potentially help alleviate joint discomfort. Adding a sprinkle of turmeric (organic and specifically sourced for pet consumption) to your pet's food, or incorporating curcumin supplements formulated for pets, might offer some relief.

**Remember:** Herbs are not a replacement for veterinary treatment for age-related conditions. Always consult your veterinarian before introducing any new herbs into your pet's routine, and ensure they are safe for senior pets.

## DIY Delights for Discerning Senior Pallets: Recipes and Remedies Tailored for Age

Just because your pet is a senior doesn't mean they can't enjoy delicious and nutritious treats! Here are a few recipe ideas that are gentle on their digestive systems and cater to their changing needs:

**Senior Superfood Smoothie:**

- 1 cup unsweetened applesauce
- 1/2 cup plain, low-fat yogurt
- 1/4 cup frozen blueberries
- 1 tablespoon pumpkin puree

- 1 teaspoon ground flaxseed

This power-packed smoothie is a fantastic source of antioxidants, fiber, and probiotics, all beneficial for senior pets. Simply blend all the ingredients together until smooth, and offer it to your senior companion in a shallow bowl or lick mat.

**Golden Oldie Gravy for Enhanced Appetite:**

- 1 cup low-sodium chicken broth
- 1 tablespoon cooked, mashed sweet potato
- 1/2 teaspoon turmeric (organic and pet-safe)
- Pinch of freshly ground ginger

This flavorful gravy can be poured over your pet's regular kibble to entice them to eat, especially if they're experiencing a decreased appetite due to age. The warmth and aroma of the gravy can be particularly appealing to senior pets.

**Remember:** These are just a few ideas to get you started. As you explore the world of senior pet care, you'll discover a vast array of other delicious and nutritious ingredients you can incorporate into your pet's diet. Always prioritize safety by consulting your veterinarian before introducing any new foods or supplements.

## Preventative Care: The Cornerstone of a Long and Healthy Senior Life

While herbs and homemade treats can play a supportive role, proactive preventative care is the cornerstone of a long and healthy senior life for your pet. Here's how Here's how proactive preventative care can benefit your senior pet:

- **Nutritional Support:** As our pets age, their dietary needs change. Senior pets often require food that is lower in calories but still rich in essential nutrients. Discuss with your veterinarian the possibility of switching your senior companion to a high-quality diet specifically formulated for their age group. These diets often prioritize easily digestible ingredients, protein sources that support muscle mass (crucial for maintaining mobility), and omega-3 fatty acids which possess anti-inflammatory properties.

**Remember:** Not all commercially available "senior" pet foods are created equal. Work with your veterinarian to choose a diet that addresses your pet's specific needs and preferences.

- **Routine Wellness Exams:** Scheduling regular wellness exams with your veterinarian is crucial for early detection of any age-related health concerns. These exams typically involve a physical examination, bloodwork, and potentially other diagnostic tests depending on your pet's individual needs. Early detection and intervention can significantly improve the prognosis for many age-related conditions, ensuring your senior pet enjoys a longer and healthier life.

**Think of it this way:** Regular wellness exams are like preventative maintenance for your pet's health. Just like you wouldn't wait for your car to break down before taking it for an oil change, don't wait for your pet to exhibit obvious signs of illness before scheduling a checkup.

- **Dental Care:** Dental health is crucial for overall well-being, and this is especially true for senior pets. Regular dental cleanings performed by your veterinarian can help prevent periodontal disease, a painful condition that can affect not only your pet's mouth but also their overall health. Additionally, brushing your senior pet's teeth at home with a pet-specific toothpaste can help maintain good oral hygiene and prevent the buildup of plaque and tartar.

- **Weight Management:** Obesity can exacerbate joint pain and strain vital organs in senior pets. If your senior companion is overweight, work with your veterinarian to develop a safe and gradual weight loss plan. This might involve slight adjustments to portion sizes, increased exercise opportunities tailored to their abilities, or switching to a weight-management diet formulated for senior pets.

By incorporating these preventative care measures into your senior pet's routine, you're not just adding years to their life, you're adding life to their years. They'll enjoy a higher quality of life, with more energy, less discomfort, and a greater ability to participate in activities they love.

**Remember:** Every senior pet is an individual, and their needs will vary. Open communication with your veterinarian is key to tailoring a preventative care plan that addresses your pet's specific health status and promotes their overall well-being. Don't hesitate to ask questions, voice your concerns, and work collaboratively with your veterinary team to ensure your cherished senior companion enjoys a comfortable and enriching golden age.

## Living Life to the Fullest: Enriching the Golden Years

Senior pets may not have the boundless energy of their youth, but that doesn't mean their lives can't be filled with joy, love, and enriching experiences. Here are some tips to make their golden years truly golden:

- **Adjusting Activities:** Senior pets might not be able to keep up with the same level of exercise they enjoyed in their younger years. However, gentle walks, playtime with favorite toys, or even short swimming sessions (if your pet enjoys water) can all contribute to their physical and mental well-being. Tailor activities to their current capabilities and adjust the intensity and duration as needed.

- **Mental Stimulation:** Just like physical exercise, mental stimulation is crucial for senior pets. Interactive toys that challenge them to problem-solve, food puzzles that dispense treats as they work for them, and even basic obedience training sessions (kept short and positive) can all help keep their minds sharp and engaged.

- **Creating a Comforting Environment:** As pets age, their eyesight and hearing might deteriorate. Make their environment safe and familiar by keeping furniture arrangements consistent, providing comfortable bedding in quiet areas, and using nightlights if necessary. Additionally, avoid introducing new pets or making significant changes to their routine, as this can be stressful for senior companions.

- **Showering Them with Love:** Perhaps the most important aspect of senior pet care is simply showering them with love and affection. Spend quality time with them, offer them gentle petting and massages, and make them feel cherished members of the family. This connection is not only emotionally fulfilling for them, but it also strengthens the human-animal bond that you share.

By implementing these strategies, you can transform your senior pet's golden years into a time of comfort, joy, and a deep sense of connection. Remember, they've given you years of unconditional love and companionship, now it's your turn

## Chapter 8: Safety Guidelines and FAQ - Navigating the World of Herbal Remedies for Pets

In the previous chapter, we explored the exciting potential of herbal support for our furry (or feathered) companions. We delved into the wonders of plants like seaweed, nettle, and alfalfa, uncovering the ways they can contribute to our pet's overall well-being. But before diving headfirst into the world of herbal remedies, it's essential to equip ourselves with the knowledge to navigate this realm safely and effectively.

This chapter acts as your comprehensive guide to ensuring responsible herbal supplementation for your pet. We'll delve into the "dos and don'ts" of safe administration, tackling crucial topics like proper dosage, potential interactions with medications, and recognizing any signs of adverse reactions. Think of it as putting on your metaphorical safety goggles and lab coat – we're about to embark on a scientific exploration of herbal support for pets!

But knowledge isn't a one-way street. As a veterinarian, I understand that pet parents often have a multitude of questions when it comes to herbal remedies. This chapter also serves as an FAQ, addressing common concerns owners have about incorporating these natural supplements into their pet's routine.

So, whether you're a seasoned pet parent well-versed in holistic wellness, or a curious newcomer intrigued by the potential of herbal support, this chapter has something for you. Let's embark on a journey of responsible pet ownership, ensuring our beloved companions experience the potential benefits of herbal remedies while prioritizing their safety and well-being.

## The Dos and Don'ts of Safe Herbal Administration

Just like any medication, herbal supplements require a measured approach to ensure your pet benefits from their properties without experiencing any unwanted side effects. Here are some crucial "dos and don'ts" to keep in mind:

**Do:**

- **Research, Research, Research:** Before introducing any new herb into your pet's diet, conduct thorough research on its specific benefits and potential side effects. Not all herbs are suitable for all pets, and some can even be toxic to certain species. Reliable online resources from reputable veterinary organizations or consultations with a holistic veterinarian are invaluable tools for gathering accurate information.

- **Start Low, Go Slow:** When introducing a new herbal remedy, always begin with a very small dose, gradually increasing it over several days as tolerated. This allows your pet's body to adjust to the new supplement and minimizes the risk of any adverse reactions.

- **Prioritize Quality:** Just like with human food, quality matters when it comes to herbal supplements for pets. Choose reputable brands that prioritize organic ingredients and clearly state the dosage on the label. Avoid products with vague labeling or questionable sourcing practices.

- **Read the Label Carefully:** Every herbal supplement comes with a label containing crucial information like dosage recommendations, potential side effects, and any known drug interactions. Read this label thoroughly and adhere to the recommended dosage based on your pet's weight and age.

- **Work with your Veterinarian:** Never view herbal remedies as a replacement for veterinary care. Discuss your desire to incorporate these supplements into your pet's routine with your vet. They can offer valuable guidance based on your pet's individual needs and medical history, ensuring the chosen herbs are safe and won't interact with any medications your pet might be taking.

## Don't:

- **Treat "Natural" as Synonymous with Risk-Free:** Just because an herb is "natural" doesn't automatically make it safe for your pet. Certain herbs can be quite potent and even toxic in high doses or for specific species. Always research the specific herb before introducing it to your pet's diet.

- **Overdose:** Temptation might strike to "double down" on the dosage if you don't see immediate results. However, exceeding the recommended dosage can lead to serious side effects. Remember, "less is often more" when it comes to herbal remedies for pets.

- **Ignore Adverse Reactions:** Pay close attention to your pet's behavior after introducing a new herbal supplement. Signs like lethargy, vomiting, diarrhea, or unusual skin irritation could indicate an adverse reaction. If you notice any of these signs, discontinue the herb immediately and consult your veterinarian.

- **Mix and Match Without Guidance:** While combining different herbs for a synergistic effect might seem appealing, it can be a risky proposition without proper knowledge. Certain herbs can have negative interactions when combined. Consult with your veterinarian or a qualified herbalist specializing in animal care before mixing and matching herbal supplements.

- **Self-Diagnose and Treat:** Herbal remedies can be a fantastic complement to veterinary care, but they're not a substitute for it. If your pet is experiencing any health concerns, schedule an appointment with your veterinarian for a proper diagnosis and treatment plan.

*By adhering to these "dos" and "don'ts," you can ensure your pet experiences the potential benefits of herbal support in a safe and responsible manner. Now, let's delve deeper into some specific concerns that often arise when navigating the world of herbal remedies for pets.*

### Herb-Drug Interactions and Contraindications: Understanding the Potential Risks

One of the most crucial considerations when incorporating herbal supplements into your pet's routine is the potential for interactions with medications they might already be taking. Certain herbs can have a potentiating effect, meaning they can amplify the effects of medications, leading to unwanted side effects. Conversely, some herbs can actually render medications less effective.

Here's a breakdown of some common concerns:

- **Blood Thinners:** If your pet is on blood-thinning medications like warfarin, avoid herbs like garlic, ginger, and turmeric. These herbs possess natural blood-thinning properties and can interact with medications, potentially increasing the risk of bleeding.
- **Antidepressants:** St. John's Wort, a popular herbal remedy for human depression, can interact with some antidepressant medications prescribed

to pets. This interaction can lead to a condition called serotonin syndrome, which can cause tremors, agitation, and even seizures.

- **Anti-inflammatory Medications:** Nonsteroidal anti-inflammatory drugs (NSAIDs) like aspirin and carprofen are commonly used to treat pain and inflammation in pets. However, certain herbs like willow bark and devil's claw also possess anti-inflammatory properties. Combining these herbs with NSAIDs can increase the risk of stomach ulcers and other gastrointestinal issues.

**Contraindications:** Just like medications, certain herbs have contraindications, meaning they are not suitable for specific health conditions or pet demographics. For instance, milk thistle, an herb commonly used for liver support, can actually worsen liver disease in some cases. Pregnant or nursing pets may also have specific contraindications for certain herbs.

## The Importance of Consulting Your Veterinarian:

Understanding these potential interactions and contraindications reinforces the importance of discussing herbal remedies with your veterinarian before introducing them to your pet. Your veterinarian can assess your pet's individual needs and medical history, ensuring the chosen herbs are safe and won't interact with any medications your pet might be taking.

They can also recommend the appropriate dosage based on your pet's specific needs and provide guidance on the best way to introduce the new supplement into their routine. Remember, your veterinarian is your trusted partner in your pet's well-being, and their expertise is invaluable when navigating the complexities of herbal support.

## Common Questions from Pet Parents: Addressing Your Concerns

As a veterinarian, I understand that pet parents often have a multitude of questions when it comes to herbal remedies. Here, we'll address some of the most frequently asked questions to empower you to make informed decisions about incorporating these natural supplements into your pet's life:

- **Can herbal remedies replace my pet's regular medications?**

Herbal remedies should be viewed as complementary to traditional veterinary medicine, not a replacement for it. If your pet has a diagnosed health condition, it's crucial to continue their prescribed medications and follow your veterinarian's treatment plan. Herbal remedies can offer additional support for specific concerns, but they are not a cure-all.

- **How long will it take to see results from herbal remedies?**

Unlike medications with immediate effects, herbal remedies often take time to work their magic. Be patient and consistent with administration. Depending on the specific herb and the desired outcome, it could take several weeks to notice any changes in your pet's health.

- **What are some signs my pet might be having an adverse reaction to an herbal supplement?**

Common signs of an adverse reaction include vomiting, diarrhea, lethargy, loss of appetite, or unusual skin irritation. If you notice any of these signs after introducing a new herbal remedy, discontinue it immediately and consult your veterinarian.

- **Where can I buy high-quality herbal supplements for my pet?**

Look for reputable pet stores or online retailers that prioritize organic ingredients and clearly state the dosage information on the label. Avoid products with vague labeling or questionable sourcing practices. Consulting your veterinarian or a qualified herbalist can also be a valuable resource for finding high-quality herbal supplements for your pet.

- **I'm overwhelmed by the sheer number of herbal remedies available. How do I choose the right one for my pet?**

Don't feel pressured to navigate this alone! Schedule a consultation with your veterinarian or a qualified animal herbalist. They can offer personalized recommendations based on your pet's specific needs and medical history.

By understanding the "dos and don'ts" of safe herbal administration, potential herb-drug interactions, and addressing common concerns, you can confidently embark on a journey of exploring the potential benefits of herbal

# Bonus Chapter

# Herbs For Pets

*F*or better clarity here are some herbs for your pets.

1. **Chamomile:** Soothes digestive issues and anxiety. Can be given as a tea (cooled) or in capsule form.

2. **Echinacea:** Boosts the immune system. Available in tincture or capsule form.

3. **Ginger:** Relieves nausea and aids digestion. Can be given fresh, dried, or in capsule form.

4. **Valerian:** Calms anxiety and promotes relaxation. Often given in tincture form.

5. **Milk Thistle:** Supports liver health. Usually administered in capsule or tincture form.

6. **St. John's Wort:** Helps with mild depression and anxiety. Available in capsule or tincture form.

7. **Peppermint:** Soothes digestive issues and freshens breath. Can be given fresh or dried.

8. **Licorice Root:** Helps with respiratory issues and digestive discomfort. Usually administered in capsule or tincture form.

9. **Nettle:** Supports joint health and can aid in allergy relief. Often given in dried form or as a tea.

10. **Turmeric:** Anti-inflammatory properties, good for joint health. Can be given as a powder mixed with food.

11. **Saw Palmetto:** Supports urinary tract health. Usually administered in capsule form.

12. **Ginseng:** Boosts energy and supports immune function. Available in capsule or tincture form.

13. **Dandelion:** Supports liver and kidney health. Can be given fresh or dried, or as a tincture.

14. **Garlic:** Has antibacterial and antifungal properties. Should be used in moderation and only in specific formulations for pets.

15. **Oregano:** Has antibacterial properties and supports digestion. Can be given fresh or dried, or as an oil.

16. Arnica: Used topically for pain relief and to reduce inflammation. Available in cream or gel form.

17. **Marshmallow Root**: Soothes digestive issues and can help with skin irritations. Often given as a tea or in capsule form.

18. **Ashwagandha**: Adaptogenic herb that can help with stress and anxiety. Usually administered in capsule or tincture form.

19. **Burdock Root**: Supports liver health and can help with skin conditions. Can be given as a tea, capsule, or tincture.

20. **Devil's Claw**: Natural anti-inflammatory for joint pain. Available in capsule or tincture form.

21. **Cat's Claw**: Supports immune function and has anti-inflammatory

properties. Often given in capsule or tincture form.

22. **Passionflower**: Calms nervousness and anxiety. Available in tincture or capsule form.

23. **Hawthorn**: Supports heart health and circulation. Often given in capsule or tincture form.

24. **Lemon Balm**: Calming herbs that can help with anxiety and insomnia. Often given as a tea or in capsule form.

25. **Skullcap**: Helps with nervousness and excitability. Usually administered in tincture form.

26. **Slippery Elm**: Soothes digestive issues and can help with diarrhea. Often given as a powder mixed with water.

27. **Yarrow**: Stops bleeding and has antimicrobial properties. Can be used topically or given as a tea.

28. **Red Clover**: Supports skin health and can help with respiratory issues. Often given as a tea or in capsule form.

29. **Rosemary**: Supports digestion and can help with arthritis pain. Can be given fresh or dried, or as an oil.

30. **Sage**: Supports oral health and can help with digestion. Can be given fresh or dried, or as a tea.

31. **Thyme**: Supports respiratory health and has antibacterial properties. Can be given fresh or dried, or as a tea.

32. **Fennel**: Relieves gas and bloating. Can be given fresh or dried, or as a tea.

33. **Mullein**: Supports respiratory health and can help with coughing. Often given as a tea or in capsule form.

34. **Ginkgo Biloba**: Supports cognitive function and circulation. Usually administered in capsule or tincture form.

35. **Astragalus**: Boosts immune function and supports overall vitality. Often given in capsule or tincture form.

36. **Black Cohosh**: Supports hormonal balance and can help with arthritis pain.

Usually administered in capsule or tincture form.

37. **Bilberry**: Supports eye health and can help with vision problems. Often given in capsule or tincture form.

38. **Kava Kava**: Relieves anxiety and promotes relaxation. Usually administered in capsule or tincture form.

39. **Feverfew**: Natural pain reliever, particularly for headaches. Often given in capsule or tincture form.

40. **Bromelain**: Enzyme that supports joint health and reduces inflammation. Usually administered in capsule form.

41. **Chaste Tree**: Supports hormonal balance, particularly in female animals. Usually administered in capsule or tincture form.

42. **Gotu Kola**: Supports skin health and wound healing. Often given in capsule or tincture form.

43. **Horse Chestnut**: Supports circulation and can help with varicose veins.

Usually administered in capsule or tincture form.

44. **Juniper Berry**: Supports urinary tract health and can help with bladder infections. Often given in capsule or tincture form.

45. **Maca Root**: Supports energy and hormone balance. Often given in capsule or tincture form.

46. **Parsley**: Supports kidney health and freshens breath. Can be given fresh or dried, or as a tea.

47. **Raspberry Leaf**: Supports female reproductive health and can help with labor in pregnant animals. Often given as a tea or in capsule form.

48. **Schisandra**: Adaptogenic herb that supports liver health and reduces stress. Usually administered in capsule or tincture form.

49. **Uva Ursi**: Supports urinary tract health and can help with bladder infections. Often given in capsule or tincture form.

50. **White Willow Bark**: Natural pain reliever for arthritis and other inflammatory conditions. Usually administered in capsule or tincture form.

As always, it's important to consult with a veterinarian before administering any herbal remedies to your pets, as individual needs and potential interactions can vary.

# Conclusion

## A Journey of Partnership: The Legacy of Herbal Wellness for Pets

*As we reach the final chapter of this exploration into the world of herbal medicine for pets, reflect on the journey we've embarked on together. You've gained valuable knowledge on the potential benefits of herbs, learned about safe and responsible administration, and explored the importance of collaboration with your veterinarian.*

*Remember, this book isn't an ending, but rather the beginning of a transformative journey towards your pet's optimal health. As you continue exploring natural wellness options for your furry (or feathered) companion, here are some key takeaways to keep in mind:*

- ***Knowledge is Power:*** *The information you've gained empowers you to ask informed questions about your pet's health and explore natural solutions alongside your veterinarian. Continue to learn and stay updated on the evolving field of herbal medicine for pets.*

- ***Respect the Rhythm of Nature:*** *Herbs are not instant fixes. Their effectiveness often relies on consistent administration and a holistic approach to your pet's well-being. Be patient, and observant, and celebrate even the subtle improvements in your pet's health.*

- ***Quality Matters:*** *When choosing herbal remedies, opt for reputable brands that prioritize quality control and organic ingredients. Don't be afraid to ask your veterinarian for recommendations on trusted sources.*

- ***The Power of Partnership:*** *Your veterinarian is your most valuable ally in your pet's healthcare journey. Communicate openly with them about your interest in herbal remedies, and work together to create a personalized approach that considers your pet's unique needs and medical history.*

- ***Celebrate the Journey:*** *Witnessing your pet thrive on a combination of conventional veterinary care and natural support is a beautiful reward. Take joy in the small victories, celebrate* *improvements in their overall well-being, and cherish the deepening bond you share.*

*As you move forward, remember that your dedication and proactive approach to your pet's health holds immense power. By embracing the wisdom of nature, complementing it with veterinary expertise, and showering your pet with love and care, you create a foundation for a long and happy life together.*

### *The Legacy of Herbal Wellness for Pets*

*The world of herbal medicine for pets holds immense potential. As research continues and our understanding of plant-based remedies expands, the possibilities for promoting pet wellness naturally continue to blossom. This book serves as a stepping stone on this exciting journey.*

*By empowering pet owners with knowledge and fostering collaboration with veterinarians, we can collectively create a future where natural options seamlessly integrate into mainstream pet healthcare. Imagine a world where pets thrive not just from conventional medicine, but also from the gentle touch of nature's wisdom.*

***It starts with you.*** *Become an advocate for your pet's natural wellness. Share your knowledge with other pet owners. Support companies committed to ethical and sustainable sourcing of herbal remedies. Together, we can build a legacy of herbal wellness for pets, ensuring a future where nature's bounty enhances the lives of our beloved companions for generations to come.*

*The final page may be turned, but the journey continues. Embrace the power of natural wellness, cherish the bond you share with your pet, and let this be the beginning of a lifetime of holistic health and happiness for your furry (or feathered) family member.*

## The Encyclopedia of Herbal Medicine for Pets: Index

**A**

- Aloe vera (benefits, cautions for pets)
- Anise (uses, safety considerations)
- Anxiety (herbal remedies for dogs, cats)
- Arthritis (herbal support for dogs, and horses)
- Asthma (herbal options for cats, and exotic animals)

**B**

- Bladder problems (urinary tract support with herbs)
- Bloating (herbal remedies for dogs)

**C**

- Calendula (wound healing properties, safe use for pets)

- Chamomile (calming effects, uses for dogs, cats)

- Coat health (herbal support for promoting healthy fur)

- Colic (herbal remedies for horses)

- Constipation (herbal solutions for dogs, cats)

**D**

- Dandelion (liver support benefits, cautions for pets)

- Diarrhea (herbal remedies for managing loose stools)

- Digestive issues (herbal support for various digestive problems)

**E**

- Echinacea (immune system support with herbs)

- Elderberry (uses for respiratory issues, safety considerations)

- Epilepsy (herbal support alongside veterinary treatment, caution advised)

- Exotic animals (herbal remedies for specific species)

**F**

- Flea and tick control (natural approaches using herbs, consult veterinarian)

**G**

- Ginkgo biloba (cognitive function support, potential herb-drug interactions)

**H**

- Hawthorn berry (heart health support with herbs, consult veterinarian)
- Horses (herbal remedies for common equine health concerns)

I

- Immune system support (herbal options for various species)

K

- Kidney problems (herbal support for kidney health)

L

- Lavender (calming properties, safe use for pets)
- Liver support (herbal remedies for promoting liver function)

**M**

- Mange (herbal options alongside veterinary treatment)
- Milk thistle (liver support benefits, potential interactions with medications)

**N**

- Nausea (herbal remedies for managing nausea in pets)

**O**

- Oatmeal baths (soothing properties for skin irritation)

**P**

- Pain management (consult veterinarian, limited role for herbs in pain relief)

- Parasites (natural approaches alongside veterinary parasite control)

**Q**

**R**

- Respiratory issues (herbal options for supporting respiratory health)

**S**

- Skin problems (herbal remedies for addressing various skin conditions)
- Stress (herbal support for managing stress in pets)

**T**

- Ticks and fleas (natural approaches using herbs, consult veterinarian)

**U**

- Urinary tract infections (UTIs) (herbal support for urinary tract health)

**V**

- Veterinarian consultation (importance of consulting your veterinarian before using herbal remedies)

**W**

- Wound healing (herbal support for wound healing, consult veterinarian)

**X**

**Y**

**Z**

www.ingramcontent.com/pod-product-compliance
Lightning Source LLC
Chambersburg PA
CBHW061029250726
48653CB00001B/16